Decision-Making in Nursing

Thoughtful Approaches for Practice

Sandra B. Lewenson, EdD, RN, FAAN

Professor of Nursing
Lienhard School of Nursing
Pace University
Pleasantville, New York

Marie Truglio-Londrigan, PhD, RN, GNP

Professor of Nursing
Lienhard School of Nursing
Pace University
Pleasantville, New York

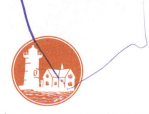

JONES AND BARTLETT PUBLISHERS

Sudbury, Massachusetts

BOSTON   TORONTO   LONDON   SINGAPORE

World Headquarters

Jones and Bartlett Publishers
40 Tall Pine Drive
Sudbury, MA 01776
978-443-5000
info@jbpub.com
www.jbpub.com

Jones and Bartlett Publishers Canada
6339 Ormindale Way
Mississauga, Ontario L5V 1J2
Canada

Jones and Bartlett Publishers
International
Barb House, Barb Mews
London W6 7PA
United Kingdom

Jones and Bartlett's books and products are available through most bookstores and online booksellers. To contact Jones and Bartlett Publishers directly, call 800-832-0034, fax 978-443-8000, or visit our website www.jbpub.com.

Substantial discounts on bulk quantities of Jones and Bartlett's publications are available to corporations, professional associations, and other qualified organizations. For details and specific discount information, contact the special sales department at Jones and Bartlett via the above contact information or send an email to specialsales@jbpub.com.

The authors, editor, and publisher have made every effort to provide accurate information. However, they are not responsible for errors, omissions, or for any outcomes related to the use of the contents of this book and take no responsibility for the use of the products and procedures described. Treatments and side effects described in this book may not be applicable to all people; likewise, some people may require a dose or experience a side effect that is not described herein. Drugs and medical devices are discussed that may have limited availability controlled by the Food and Drug Administration (FDA) for use only in a research study or clinical trial. Research, clinical practice, and government regulations often change the accepted standard in this field. When consideration is being given to use of any drug in the clinical setting, the health care provider or reader is responsible for determining FDA status of the drug, reading the package insert, and reviewing prescribing information for the most up-to-date recommendations on dose, precautions, and contraindications, and determining the appropriate usage for the product. This is especially important in the case of drugs that are new or seldom used.

Production Credits
Executive Editor: Kevin Sullivan
Acquisitions Editor: Emily Ekle
Associate Editor: Amy Sibley
Editorial Assistant: Patricia Donnelly
Production Director: Amy Rose
Production Editor: Carolyn F. Rogers
Senior Marketing Manager: Katrina Gosek
Associate Marketing Manager: Rebecca Wasley
Manufacturing and Inventory Coordinator: Amy Bacus
Composition: Paw Print Media
Cover Design: Kristin E. Ohlin
Cover Image: © Jong Kiam Soon/ShutterStock, Inc.
Printing and Binding: Malloy, Inc.
Cover Printing: Malloy, Inc.

Library of Congress Cataloging-in-Publication Data
Decision-making in nursing : thoughtful approaches for practice
[edited by] Sandra B. Lewenson, Marie Truglio-Londrigan.
    p. ; cm.
  Includes bibliographical references and index.
  ISBN-13: 978-0-7637-4435-9 (pbk.)
  ISBN-10: 0-7637-4435-2 (pbk.)
  1. Nursing--Decision making. I. Lewenson, Sandra. II.
Truglio-Londrigan, Marie.
  [DNLM: 1. Decision Making. 2. Nursing Care—methods. WY 100 D294
2008]
  RT42.D433 2008
  610.73—dc22
                              2007031565
6048

Printed in the United States of America
11 10 09 08 07   10 9 8 7 6 5 4 3 2 1

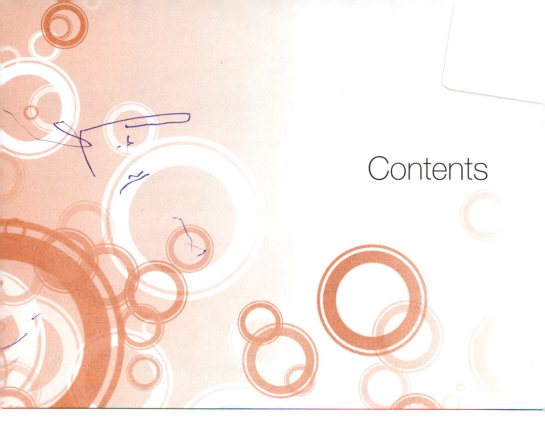

Contents

Chapter 1 Know Yourself: Reflective Decision-Making 1

Marie Truglio-Londrigan and Sandra B. Lewenson

Chapter 7 Media and Decision-Making 105
Sandy Summers and Harry Jacobs Summers

Chapter 8 Flattening the Field: Group Decision-Making 131
Marie Truglio-Londrigan

Chapter 9 Evidence-Based Decision-Making 145
Christine Pintz

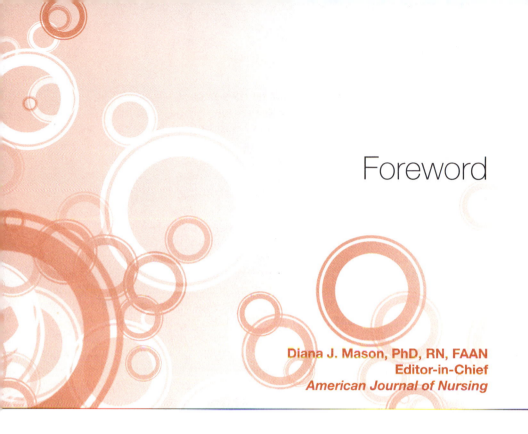

Foreword

Diana J. Mason, PhD, RN, FAAN
Editor-in-Chief
American Journal of Nursing

By all accounts, Julie Thao was an excellent, veteran obstetrics nurse, yet her decisions on July 4 and 5, 2006, led to the death of Jasmine Gant, a 16-year-old laboring woman; the loss of her job; the loss of her license; and a felony charge for "criminal neglect of a patient causing great bodily harm" that later was reduced to two misdemeanors. Her errors included:

- Not ensuring that the patient had the regulation, bar-coded wristband in place
- Failing to use the 3-week-old medication bar-coding system that could have alerted her to the fact that she was about to give Gant an unordered epidural (bupivacaine) medication instead of IV penicillin
- Failing to review the five rights of medication administration before giving the wrong medication the wrong route (bupivacaine IV)

Why would a veteran nurse make such decisions?

Thao's worst decision was the one she made on July 4 to work a double shift, sleep for less than 8 hours at the hospital, and then work another shift. When she made the errors, she had worked about 20 hours in a 28-hour period. We know that fatigue is associated with an increased risk of errors; that too many nurses are working too many hours, impairing their judgment, and putting the lives and well-being of their patients in jeopardy (Rogers, Hwang, Scott, Aiken, & Dinges, 2004; Trinkoff, Geiger-Brown, Brady, Lipscomb, & Muntaner, 2006).

Perhaps she agreed to work these hours because she wasn't aware of this literature that documents an increased risk of errors once one exceeds 12 hours in a 24-hour period. Too many nurses believe that their education stops with the original program that led to their license—they don't pursue higher degrees or even read nursing journals (Mason, 2007a; Bevill, Lacey, & Cleary, 2007)—raising questions about the meaning of "informed" decision-making.

Or maybe she thought herself invulnerable. She probably had worked many double shifts in her 16 years of nursing practice—and I've argued elsewhere (Mason, 2007b) that Thao was probably seen as a "good" nurse—the one who will do those double shifts when the hospital is understaffed. I don't know Julie Thao but she may come from a family or culture that values a work ethic in which one should go to whatever lengths necessary to be the "good" (translated, compliant, and unchallenging) employee.

However, to put the blame of the errors on the shoulders of Julie Thao is a disservice to her and to the memory of Jasmine Gant. Thao and nurses like her are working in systems that too often fail to value nursing care as the core business of institutions. People rarely become patients in hospitals if they don't need nursing care. Despite a substantial and growing body of research documenting the link between nurse staffing and both clinical and financial outcomes of care, hospitals and other health care organizations continue to expect nurses to care for too many patients and fail to put into place the policies and systems that will catch the errors that all of us make ("to err is human") and support thoughtful decision-making by frontline clinicians. Hospitals may ignore the research on nurse staffing while investing in expensive, high-tech diagnostic equipment, for example. In a provocative editorial in *Nursing Research*, Blegen (2006) challenges us to carefully examine the decisions that are being made in the name of patient safety and quality improvement. For example, she notes that hospitals and other health care facilities are paying for expensive, high-tech solutions to patient safety such as bar-coding systems while failing to pay for the systems and support necessary for collecting standardized data on nurse-sensitive outcomes or investing in improving communication among providers or with patients that could markedly reduce errors and improve the quality of care.

Health care organizations are run by people who are making decisions that can either cultivate or undermine conditions and systems that are conducive to safe, humane care. Why does a chief nurse officer (CNO) fail to advocate for better staffing when she or he knows that poor staffing can lead to a higher rate of deaths and complications, as well as be costly? Why does the CNO staff the hospital or home care agency by expecting or mandating overtime from existing staff? Why does the chief executive officer (CEO) expect the CNO to staff at current levels despite the increased acuity of patients and higher census? Why does the CEO think it is more important to invest in high-tech diagnostic equipment than in nursing personnel? Why does the chief medical officer insist on putting into place "rapid response" teams to try to reduce cardiac arrests and morality instead of insisting on adequate staffing and staff development to prevent the need for such teams (Winters, Pham, & Pronovost, 2006)?

Administrators struggle with such decisions for a variety of reasons, but chief among them are decisions made by policy makers. Why do Medicare and private insurers pay for disease diagnosis and treatment but lump nursing care into room charges, putting nurses at a distinct disadvantage when trying to make the business case for better staffing (Welton, 2006; Welton, Zone-Smith, & Fischer, 2006)? Why are policy makers talking only about how to cover the uninsured by finding ways to extend payment for current models of health care rather than thinking about providing all people with a model of care that focuses on prevention, health promotion, and the patient's and family's goals and priorities for care, as already exists in hospice and palliative care?

Current practice and policy decisions of nurses, administrators, and policy makers are grounded in history, as is noted in this book. For example, in Chapter 2, Lewenson writes about the historic dominance of medicine to the extent that nursing knowledge was obscured until Lavinia Dock wrote about uniquely nursing practices. Today's nurses continue to struggle with medical dominance; a dominance that was codified when the first medical practice acts were written. These acts included a scope of practice for physicians that covered all of health care, leaving nurses and other providers to continually fight to carve out legal scopes of practice that enable them to provide care without physician supervision (Safriet, 1994). Thus, we make decisions that reflect an insecurity about our right and ability to own our knowledge, even when it might benefit patients.

In an era of evidence-based practice, we often assume that the "evidence" is truth and can guide our practice. However, Ioannidis (2005) and others (Deyo, Psaty, Simon, Wagner, & Omenn, 1997) have argued that even the decisions of researchers about what to study and how to study it can be manipulated by funders and other groups that may have a vested in the outcomes of the research, as well as the researcher's own aspirations. "Publish or perish" becomes an academic albatross when journals are reluctant to publish studies that fail to find positive results, leading some researchers to commit fraud and scientific misconduct. Furthermore, what high level of evidence for practice do we have? Funding for nursing research pales beside the funding of the pharmaceutical industry and even the National Institutes of Health (NIH). In 2006, the National Institute for Nursing Research received a paltry $137 million out of a budget of $28.8 billion for all of the NIH. This is yet another example of the importance of public policy to nurses' clinical decision-making. If clinicians are expected to engage in evidence-based practice, what happens to clinical decision-making when the only available randomized clinical trials are of pharmaceutical interventions for conditions or health problems that nursing experiences indicate are responsive to nonpharmaceutical approaches? These issues and questions suggest that nurses must be thoughtful about their reliance on "evidence-based" guidelines for care and be critical consumers of research and other "best practice" evidence.

While each of us has a responsibility to make thoughtful decisions about the care we're providing to patients and their families, we also must make thoughtful decisions and speak out about the larger issues and policies that shape the context in which our decisions are make. We must examine why we are content to be invisible within our institutions and in society. Why do we speak out-or not-about poor or unsafe working conditions? Why do we continue to work in institutions that we know are unsafe? The decision to speak out or to walk out is itself worthy of examination by each of us. What is our comfort level with living up to the advocacy role almost all nurses espouse? If we're uncomfortable with challenging the status quo and leading change, why? In this book, Elizabeth Furlong suggests that nurses ask themselves, "How did I spend my time?"; "Did I spend it justly?"; and "Is it just (to patients and to oneself) to continue working in an environment where there is consistent mandatory overtime?"

In Chapter 4 of this book, Joy Buck tells the story of Kate, who left hospital practice because her staff colleagues refused to respect the wishes of a patient and his wife at the end of life. I was moved by this story of one nurse fighting a whole system of values and priorities that resulted in care that was inhumane. Buck speaks about the moral distress that such situations create in nurses who know there is a better way to care but suppress their own and nursing's values to survive in systems that are dominated by an ethic of cure at the expense of an ethic of care. Still, nurses such as Kate beginning to refuse to tolerate systems of care in which such moral distress is rampant and unaddressed. The nursing shortage is created in part by a failure of an ethic of care to prevail in our health care organizations and to be supported by public policies that support professional caregiving.

There are hospitals and home care agencies and long-term care facilities and schools and ambulatory care centers that provide supportive work environments and excellent, safe systems of care that are truly family and patient centered. They are headed by visionary, thoughtful decision-makers who support the development and implementation of thoughtful decision-making by their staff. These are proactive, risk-taking innovators who relish the challenge of making decisions that are in the best interests of the people they serve, whether staff or patients. We all need to learn from such role models of excellent decision-making and to examine our own decisions that support either the spread of such centers of excellence or the perpetuation of mediocrity and outright bad, unsafe care.

We are all Julie Thao. We make decisions that aren't always logical or beneficial to ourselves or our patients despite our best intentions. We are products of our own genetic make up, familial values, cultural and sociopolitical contexts, and historical precedent—but perhaps we can make better decisions if we reflect on how and why we make decisions. This book provides nurses with a guide for examining who we are, some of the contextual factors that shape our decision-making, and the role of public policy in macro-level decision-making. I was stunned by Lewenson's and Truglio-Londrigan's revelation in the preface that there have been no other books examining nurses' decision-making. *Decision-Making in Nursing: Thoughtful Approaches for Practice* is long overdue. I hope it will serve as a foundation for future works and will help each of us to examine why we make the decisions we do— whether in service to our individual patients, our workplaces, our society, or ourselves.

References

Bevill, J., Lacey, L., & Cleary, B. (2007). Educational mobility of RNs in North Carolina: Who will teach tomorrow's nurses? *American Journal of Nursing, 107*(5), 60–70.

Blegen, M. (2006). Safety of healthcare: An amazing possibility. *Nursing Research, 55*(5), 299.

Deyo, R.A., Psaty, B.M., Simon, G., Wagner, E.H., & Omenn, G.S. (1997). The messenger under attack-Intimidation of researchers by special-interest groups. *New England Journal of Medicine, 336*(16), 1176–1180.

Ioannidis, J. (2005). Contradicted and initially stronger effects in highly cited clinical research. *Journal of the American Medical Association, 294*(2), 218–228.

Mason, D. J. (2007a). Which nurse do you want? *American Journal of Nursing,* 107(5), 11.

Mason, D. J. (2007b). Good nurse-Bad nurse: Is it an error or crime? *American Journal of Nursing,* 107(3), 11.

Rogers, A.E., Hwang, W.T., Scott, L.D., Aiken, L.H., & Dinges, D.F. (2004). The working hours of hospital staff nurses and patient safety. *Health Affairs,* 23(4), 202–212.

Safriet, B. (1994). Impediments to progress in health care workforce policy: License and practice laws. *Inquiry,* 31(30), 310–317.

Trinkoff, A., Geiger-Brown, J., Brady, B., Lipscomb, J., Muntaner, C. (2006). How long and how much are nurses now working? *American Journal of Nursing,* 106(4), 60–71.

Welton, J. (2006). Paying for nursing care in hospitals. *American Journal of Nursing,* 106(11), 67–69.

Welton, J.M., Zone-Smith, L., & Fischer, M.H. (2006). Adjustment of inpatient care reimbursement for nursing intensity. *Policy, Politics, and Nursing Practice,* 7(4), 270–280.

Winters, B., Pham, J., & Pronovost, P. (2006). Rapid response teams-Walk, don't run. *Journal of the American Medical Association,* 296(13), 1645–1647.

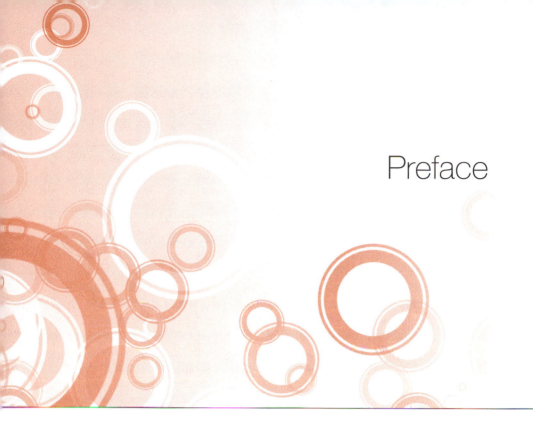

Preface

Making decisions in the twenty-first century requires reflective thought, interdisciplinary focus, global perspectives, use of technology, and comfort with ambiguity. Nurses face challenges every day when caring for people. A choice for one person may not be the appropriate one for another. Factors such as diverse populations, changing health care systems, limited resources, and a challenging environment provide some of the reasons why we must look at the different ways we make decisions. Nurses need to critically think through their decisions, be willing to be flexible, and know what they know and what they do not know, as well as be aware of many ways to approach a decision. Nurses need to be reflective of who they are in the context of their patients, families, and communities.

Decision-Making in Nursing explores the contributions of a variety of decision-making approaches that add to the ways of knowing and the evidence that enables nursing professionals to be reflective, critical, flexible, and comfortable with the many decisions they make on a daily basis. This book offers a variety of thoughtful approaches that the practitioner may integrate in their practice. The book looks at the various ways in which we make decisions and shows that although the various approaches may be presented independently, they are interdependently connected. Carper (1992) recognized that the various "patterns of knowing" are "not mutually exclusive" and described them as "interrelated and interdependent" (p.77). We view the various approaches in a similar manner. While each chapter focuses on a specific approach used in decision-making, it does so for the purpose of allowing the nurse to understand and apply the concepts of this approach in their decision.

The significance of this book lies in its reflective, multidimensional approach to decision-making. (See **Figure 1**.) We see the health care arena and the care provided as extremely complex and a dynamic process that one can imagine as a "holographic" view of the experience at any given point in time. Depending on the angle you are looking at, the holographic image changes. Nurses looking at a patient, family, or community may need to choose a different decision-making approach based upon the multidimensional image that is presented at any given moment. Nurses, therefore, must be aware of the many ways in which decisions can be made and implemented in the care of individuals,

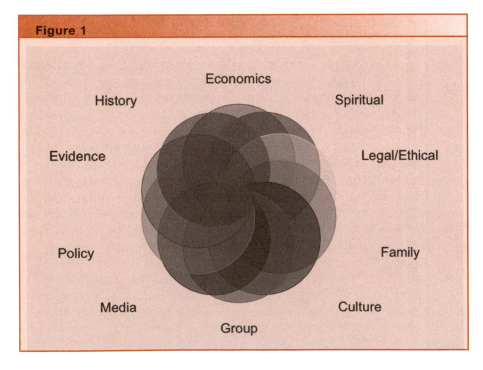

Figure 1

Economics

History

Spiritual

Evidence

Legal/Ethical

Policy

Family

Media

Culture

Group

families, and communities. Nurses require the ability to be fluid in their thinking, which enables them to see and be willing to look at the issues in front of them from different vantage points.

Nurses who practice with a one-dimensional approach to care frequently find their outcomes limited and inconsistent with the philosophical beliefs of nursing. For example, nurses in a county department of health identified that the morbidity and mortality statistics rates for prostate cancer in black males to be alarmingly high. These nurses, along with other public health officials, dutifully developed and implemented a public health initiative for the prevention of prostate cancer including early identification and treatment for black men. Their decision to implement this program was solely based on statistical evidence and lacked depth or breadth that would have considered culture, race, ethnicity, family, history, economics, legal and ethical issues, and a myriad of other factors that may have influenced the success of this program. The program did not acknowledge these other factors and therefore failed to meet the desired health care outcomes. These nurses lacked a holistic view that nursing claims to hold. They functioned more like Benner's (1984) novice-level nurses and less like an expert who typically uses a more holistic view. Nevertheless, all nurses need to consider the various approaches that interrelate and are interdependent in their decision-making process. An awareness of the multiple approaches of decision-making would have allowed the public health nurses to expand their decision-making from just the one-model statistical approach to more of a holistic approach. By using an expanded view, they would take into account these various factors, reached out, and partnered with this targeted population and other organizations in the community who work with them. This broader partnership would have allowed the planners to see the intervention strategy in a different way and thus understand the need to expand their worldview when making decisions.

If we look at the use of restraints with the elderly, decisions were made based on what was thought to ensure the safety of the patient; however, decisions were not based on evidence such as history, patient preferences, or ethical concerns. Brush and Capezuti (2001) looked at the time hospitals first introduced side rails as intervention strategies to prevent falls. Through their historical research, they found that side rails were first used in the 1930s to prevent falls and possible lawsuits. Nurses did not have evidence nor seek evidence that supported the safety aspect of using siderails. The physical, psychological, ethical, and economic questions surrounding the use of restraints had not been addressed during this early period of time. However, today, because guidelines in care are established by the U.S. Department of Health and Human Services, evidence-based practice is the driving the force. This evidence includes not only empirical data, but also the evidence provided by the historical antecedents.

We felt that nurses needed *Decision-Making in Nursing* to provide the tools to look at the decision-making as a multidimensional reflective experience. The book examines how self-reflection, history, legal and ethical, spirituality, culture, family, media, group, evidenced-based practice, economics, and health policy affect the way we make decisions. It offers ways that nurses can use to critically think through a decision. Although other approaches to decision-making exist, we selected these as important to consider throughout the decision-making process. And although nurses may not use each one approach for every decision they make, just being aware of the possibilities allows for the complexity, fluidity, and flexibility in thinking that nurses need.

Each chapter will include at least one case study using a nursing scenario that will illustrate the use of a particular approach in an actual practice setting. We use nursing scenarios as exemplars for several reasons. Nurses represent most of the health care professionals in the United States; there are over two million nurses reported in the country. Nurses touch the lives of people—in every situation—from birth to death, in health and illness. People turn to nurses to ask questions to make better health care decisions. Nurses deal in human responses. Decisions are a human response to a particular situation. Our own background and the background of our contributors as nurses and nursing educators provide a rich tapestry from which we can draw. We use this multidimensional reflective approach to better understand the process of decision-making in the health care setting. To allow for diversity of ideas, we asked each contributor to write from their own experiences, use their own case studies (as many as they liked), and to give the readers their own thoughts on the subject they were assigned.

Chapter 1, *Know Yourself: Reflective Decision-Making*, explains the use of self-reflection in the decision-making process. Authors Marie Truglio-Londrigan and Sandy Lewenson use themselves as a "case study" in which they present a reflection of who they are and how this may have affected the decisions they have made. The self-reflection that the authors undergo also demonstrates the way they filter the logic and critical thinking that they undergo when making decisions. Like Durgahee (1996) observes, "knowledge lies within the practical situations" (p. 426). Self-reflection asks that we look at ourselves and to transform our everyday life experience to knowledge that we apply in decision-making. What the authors present is that knowledge lies embedded within everyday life experiences.

Chapter 2, titled *Looking Back: History and Decision-Making in Health Care*, discusses how history informs decisions. Author Sandra B. Lewenson looks at the "history" of decision-making in nursing and examines how nurses have made decisions in the past. It also looks at how the history of the profession itself affects decision-making in the clinical and educational arena. The role of women, modernization of hospitals, and the changing roles of health providers have influenced the kinds of decisions that have made and continue to be made. Examples of historiographical studies are used throughout the chapter to explain how important history is to decision-making. The case study used depicts a community assessment looking at historical data from 1893 and how nurses like Lillian Wald made important health care decisions on the Lower East Side of New York.

Chapter 3, *Right or Wrong: Legal and Ethical Issues and Decision-Making*, discusses the legal and ethical issues that inform the health care decision-making process. Nurse-attorney Elizabeth Furlong presents a case study showing what can happen if a proposed law in Nebraska passes and the bearing it could have on nurses' decisions regarding the care of a dying patient. The law, if it were to pass, would create tension between the nurses' professional code of ethics, the law, and their own beliefs about care. The contributor provides a discussion about the ethics of caring and how it pertains to nurses' decision-making process. In addition, this chapter looks at the factors that influence the health care professional as they make the determination to alter health care policy.

In Chapter 4, *More than Prayer: Spirituality and Decision-Making*, noted historian Joy Buck examines spirituality and the affect it has on nurses' ability to make decisions and help patients do the same. The chapter takes into account the patients' spiritual needs, the historical relevance of spirituality and nursing care, and the nurses' ability to understand their own spirituality and that of the patient, family, and community. Buck addresses values, religious beliefs, and what is meant by spirituality and decision-making in nursing. Compelling case studies throughout the chapter illustrate the need for nurses to be aware of how spirituality of the patient and their own spirituality influence the decision-making process.

Culture plays an important role in how people respond to issues surrounding sickness and health. Chapter 5, *Culture and Decision-Making*, examines the impact culture has on a nurse's decision-making ability. In this chapter, nurse educator Caroline Camuñas examines how the culture of the provider as well as the consumer affects decision-making. Camuñas presents a cogent discussion about organizational culture, various ways of knowing, and the importance of dialogue to understand culture. It also looks at how the culture of each person in the decision-making process affect the way the decision is made and how they relate to each other, as well as the decision itself. This chapter forces nurses to reflect on who they are, and in so doing, be mindful of their conduct, decisions they make, and how they relate to their patients, families, and communities.

Family plays a large role in the life of an individual and thus on the decisions surrounding health care. Chapter 6, *Who Is Family?: Family and Decision-Making*, presents three different case studies that exemplify three different families and the need for nurses to be mindful of the needs of each when working with families. Nurse educator Susan Salmond looks at how family members influence a health care decision and the need for health care providers to be aware of how their own family background experiences interfaces with that of their patients.

Chapter 7, *Media and Decision-Making*, explores the nature of media and decision-making. Founder of the Center for Nursing Advocacy Sandy Summers and coauthor Harry Jacobs Summers provide insights about media and techniques media may use that influence health care decision-making among professionals and the population-at-large. Examples of how media, including television, books, movies, the Internet, and public health campaigns, influences the decisions made about health care. Nursing images in the media such as the "Naughty Nurse," "The Battleaxe," and "The Angel" affect the way nursing decisions are viewed by various populations, including other health professionals, the people nurses serve, and nurses themselves. Nursism, or the bias toward the caring role (Lewenson, 1993), may block an acceptance of nurses' as decision-makers. Summers and Summers demonstrate how the media can influence both the consumer of health care and the health care provider in the process of reflective decision-making. They also provide useful steps that can be taken by nurses to positively influence the messages transmitted by the media.

Chapter 8, *Flattening the Field: Group Decision-Making*, explores the process of group decision-making. When individual members participate in a group, they bring their own ideas, culture, and values to the table. Although there may be a singular vision or goal that the group may wish to accomplish, the group must understand that each individual has their own ideas, values, and beliefs that must be attended to and respected in order for the group to be successful. In this chapter, Marie Truglio-Londrigan presents an interesting case study that explains group decision-making and the value it brings to the process of decision-making.

Nurses make decisions using evidence. This is not a new concept. Nurses have sought evidence through research since the days of Florence Nightingale. Nightingale's use of data to support her work during the Crimean War and Lillian Wald's use of data to support the work of the Henry Street Settlement laid the groundwork for nurses to use evidence to support their work. In Chapter 9, *Evidence-Based Decision-Making*, nurse educator Christine Pintz examines the various dimensions of evidence that nurses must gather to make informed decisions for best practice. This chapter includes the systematic reviews, quantitative and qualitative perspectives, history, patient preferences, and other sources of evidence as nurses engage in decision-making.

Many decisions regarding health care are influenced by economic reality. Nurses need to know and understand how economics drives health care decisions. The trick is how nurses use economic data to inform their decisions without comprising the other dimensions of the multidimensional reflective decision-making approaches. In Chapter 10, *Right on the Money: Economics and Decision-Making*, nursing educator Marcia E. Tyler-Evans addresses macro-level economics as a way to understand the micro-level economics that nurses face in practice. Health care providers need to understand the concepts behind economic decision-making and the ultimate outcome pertaining to care rendered to individuals, families, and populations.

In Chapter 11, *Getting Involved: Public Policy and the Decision-Making Process*, health policy consultant Judith K. Leavitt looks at how legislators make decisions, very often influenced by special interest groups and lobbyist. Nurses play an active role by providing lawmakers with knowledge and evidence necessary to make informed decisions with regard to health policy that ultimately have a direct effect on populations. Nurses especially can offer evidence that drive needed policy changes. Incorporating focused analysis of issues, community coalitions, and partnerships are all a part of this process necessary to educate and influence policy makers which is integral to health care policy decision-making.

Campbell (2004) compiled a definition of *critical thinking* from the literature as "open-minded reasoning; use of intellectual standards of reasoning including, clarity, depth and breadth of understanding and relevance of information to a situation, and questioning of assumptions and biases" (p. 195). The approaches presented in *Decision-Making in Nursing* offers nurses the tools to entertain the open-minded reasoning that critical thinking requires. The different thoughtful approaches merge as a holographic image and create a multidimensional reflective model. Imagine a holographic image as a visual of what we see as essential to use in decision-making. We also recognize that we cannot include all the infinite number of approaches that one may use in making decisions, but we have selected some that we think are important. Essential to this book is the idea that there is no one best method to use to make a decision. Using any one approach is too linear, too singular, too rigid, and too incomplete to aid nurses in the care of their patients, families, and communities in this increasingly complex world that we live. The book leaves us with more questions than answers on how to make decisions, but it gives us a way to look at the world and thus, support the work we do.

References

Benner, P. (1984). *From novice to expert: Excellence and power in clinical nursing practice.* Menlo Park: CA: Addison-Wesley.

Brush, B. L., & Capezuti, E. (2001). Historical analysis of siderail use in American hospitals. *Journal of Nursing Scholarship,* 23(4), 381–385.

Campbell, E. T. (2004). Meeting practice challenges via a clinical decision-making course. *Nurse Educator,* 29(5), 195–198.

Carper, B. A. (1992). Philosophical inquiry in nursing: An application. In J. E. Kikuchi & H. Simmons (eds.). *Philosophical inquiry in nursing* (pp. 71–80). London: Sage Publications.

Durgahee, T. (1996). Promoting reflection in post-graduate nursing: A theoretical model. *Nurse Education Today,* 16, 419–426.

Lewenson, S. B. (1993). *Taking charge: Nursing suffrage, and feminism.* New York: Garland Press.

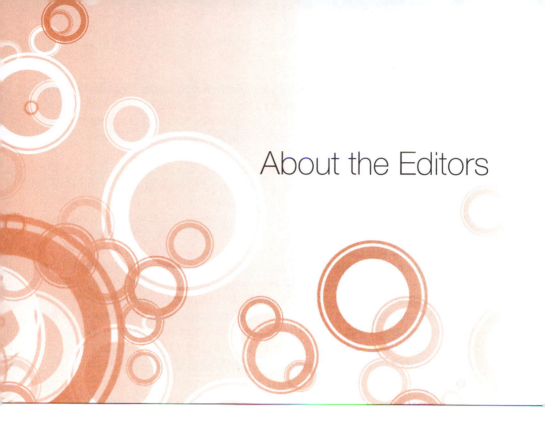

About the Editors

Sandra B. Lewenson, EdD, RN, FAAN, is a professor of nursing at the Lienhard School of Nursing, Pace University. She is a noted nurse historian and served as the president of the American Association for the History of Nursing. Dr. Lewenson teaches courses in decision-making, nursing history, and nursing education. Throughout her career, she has served in educational leadership positions, including the director of accreditation at the National League for Nursing and most recently as the associate dean for academic affairs at the Lienhard School of Nursing. Her interests include nursings' historical political activity, integrating nursing history in the curriculum, evidence of nursism and its effect on nursing recruitment and retention, and the change in nursing education from an apprenticeship model to a baccalaureate and higher degree model. She has received several awards in nursing including the Outstanding Scholarship and Research Award from the Teachers College at Columbia University, Hall of Fame of the Alumni Association of

Hunter College, the Lavinia Dock Award for Historical Scholarship and Research in Nursing, and Sigma Theta Tau's Media Nursing Print Award. She is a fellow in the American Academy of Nursing and a member of Sigma Theta Tau International Honor Society.

Marie Truglio-Londrigan, PhD, RN, GNP, has been a nurse since 1976 and primarily has practiced in community, long-term care and public health nursing. She holds a baccalaureate degree from Herbert H. Lehman College, a master's in primary health care nursing of the aged from Seton Hall University, and a doctorate in nursing from Adelphi University. Dr. Londrigan holds a faculty practice at Aging in America, Morningside House in the Bronx, New York. She has published in the areas of gerontology as well as areas pertaining to public health, health promotion and disease prevention, and ethical conduct in nursing education. Currently, Dr. Marie Truglio-Londrigan serves as a faculty member at Pace University, Lienhard School of Nursing. She is a professor and codirector of the Institute for Healthy Aging and the chair of its graduate department of nursing.

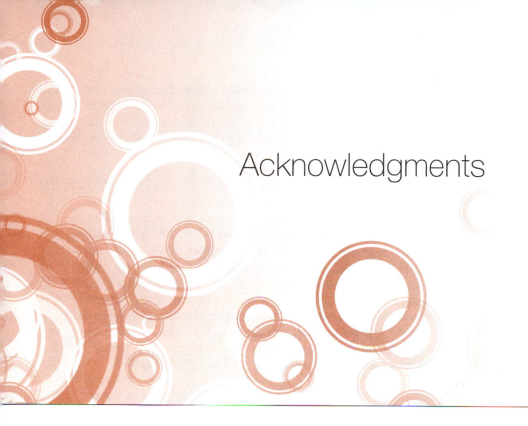

Acknowledgments

I want to acknowledge the love and support of my family who helped me think through the writing of this book and freely offered their opinions. As a family, we have had to make many life-altering decisions such as the nursing home placement for my mom, Pearl Nibur Chandler, who has Alzheimer's, and the recent move into assisted living for my 96-year-old father-in-law, George Lewenson. Each decision we made about their care brought home the relevance of this book. Thank you to Richard, my husband, for his unfailing love and support as well as ability to make clinical decisions; to my daughters Jenni and Nicky and both their terrific husbands, Chris and Jeff, who encouraged and supported me throughout all the decision-making that needed to be done both at home and in this book. We had choices and we took risks and we moved on, and for that I want to acknowledge and thank them all. I also want to acknowledge my sister, Michelle Kalina, who spent time reading, critiquing, and editing some of the chapters. Her expertise and support of my work goes above and beyond. I especially want to thank my colleague and friend, Marie Truglio-Londrigan, for her persistence and belief in this project. Finally, I want to acknowledge the wonderful graduate students who have taken the decision-making course over the past 7 years and provided us with much needed critique and ideas that have enriched this text.

Sandra B. Lewenson

Identifying that there was a need for this book was easy. The decision to actually engage in the writing process was a difficult one. Once the decision was made, there was a tremendous sense of responsibility to do the job and to do it well. There are three people in my life who have helped me in this process. They also have supported me on a daily basis just by their presence. The first is my husband Michael. Over 40 years ago, he asked me if I wanted a ride on the handles of his bicycle. I made a decision that summer day to go with him. His unwavering support has helped me ever since. Not a day goes by that I do not ask him what he thinks about certain issues and his guidance is accepted and greatly appreciated. He is my heart and my soul. To my two children, Paul and Leah, you each have taught me something in your own way. Those lessons sometimes were hard to take but I have no doubt they were lessons that I needed to learn. You both give me energy and a sense of spirit. To those who have gone before me, I thank you for providing me with memories and a solid foundation that has helped me shape a meaningful life.

Marie Truglio-Londrigan

Contributors

Joy Buck, PhD, RN
University of Pennsylvania
School of Nursing
Philadelphia, Pennsylvania

Caroline Camuñas, EdD, RN
James J. Peters Veterans Administration
  Medical Center
Bronx, New York

Elizabeth Furlong, PhD, JD, RN
Creighton University
Omaha, Nebraska

Judith K. Leavitt, MEd, RN, FAAN
Health Policy Consultant
Barnardsville, North Carolina

Christine Pintz, PhD, RN, FNP
The George Washington University
School of Medicine and Health Sciences
Washington, D.C.

Susan Salmond, EdD, RN
University of Medicine and Dentistry
School of Nursing
Newark, New Jersey

Harry Jacobs Summers, BA, JD
The Center for Nursing Advocacy
Baltimore, Maryland

Sandy Summers, MSN, MPH, RN
The Center for Nursing Advocacy
Baltimore, Maryland

Marcia E. Tyler-Evans, PhD, RN, CNAA
California State University
Bakersfield, California

Chapter 1

Know Yourself: Reflective Decision-Making

Marie Truglio-Londrigan, PhD, RN, GNP, and Sandra B. Lewenson, EdD, RN, FAAN

The genesis for this book began when we taught a graduate course in decision-making. The course, titled "Advanced Decision-Making in Primary Health Care," was one of the core courses in the graduate program at our school (O'Donnell, Lewenson, & Keith-Anderson, 2000). The course covered the various approaches to decision-making including self-reflection, history, economics, culture, family, evidence-based practice, media, group decision-making, and health care policy. These various approaches were to be used by nurses in clinical settings, but actual clinical decision-making tools were not part of this course. In preparing for the course, we found that no text existed that addressed the topics we covered in the course. After searching the literature, the faculty developed a "Course Pac" that contained the course readings; eventually we placed our readings on e-reserve.

This worked for several years, until faculty decided we wanted a more consistent way of sharing with our students and with a larger nursing audience what we had learned over time about decision-making. This required more than grouping the readings together and posting them. It required a way of translating and explaining to others what we meant by decision-making. This meant we needed to think through our thoughts on decision-making.

Self-Reflection and Decision-Making

When making decisions, nurses need to understand that decision-making requires looking inward at one's own self, then outward at the world around them, and then back in again. We understand that the decision-making process requires an understanding that the particular issue that needs a decision would often become unfocused, very much like the "holographic" image discussed in the preface of this text. As this distortion becomes evident to the decision-maker (in this instance the nurse), it is important to recognize it for what it is and to scan the environment for knowledge that helps the nurse bring the image back into focus and then a decision can be made. The process of knowledge attainment may take the many approaches that we have included in this text. The approaches included in this text—self-reflection, history, legal, ethical, spirituality, culture, family, group, evidence-based practice, economics, and health policy—are taken into account when making a decision. We wanted to codify what we were teaching about decision-making in one text that could explain our ideas.

While writing this book, the coeditors spent a great deal of time discussing decision-making. We asked ourselves: What does decision-making mean?; How can we approach it?; How can we teach students and nurses to use various approaches and strategies in their decision-making?; What have we learned from others?; and finally, What is our own "brand" or philosophical thoughts about decision-making? We both believe that in order to make meaningful decisions, a self-reflective process has to take place. Within a self-reflective process, one must examine one's own beliefs, where they come from, and what they mean. In addition, one must be able to "bracket" these beliefs (like in qualitative research) in search of answers or decisions that support care.

Self-reflection becomes an integral part of the process that allows the decision-maker to be thoughtful in the approaches used in making decisions. There is an ebb and flow of ideas that create synergy between and among the various approaches to decision-making. The synergy provides this opportunity to examine the various factors that enter into decision-making—the looking inward, outward, and then in again described earlier. The ability to understand the choices one has when making decisions and the concomitant risks that one takes with the choices selected must also be considered during the decision-making process (Buchanan & O'Connell, 2006).

Self-reflection was defined by the course faculty "as an examination of one's own thoughts and feelings, [and] requires maturity and a desire to know who you are" (O'Donnell, Lewenson, & Keith-Anderson, 2000, p. 153). We used this definition with our students and recognized that the students, many of whom were enrolled in the family nurse practitioner program, were adult learners and therefore, mature enough to examine who they were so that they could use their reflections of self to acquire and generate knowledge (Mountford & Rogers, 1996; O'Donnell, Lewenson, & Keith-Anderson, 2000).

In this first chapter, we use ourselves to explain what we mean by self-reflection and how the self-reflective process bears on decision-making. We think that by doing this we demonstrate how self-reflection may impact on decisions we make in life and how this impacts the decisions we help others make. In class we used a similar type exercise to help students reflect on their own selves and see how who they are impacts their decisions. In order to accomplish this goal, we introduce ourselves through self-reflection. We describe who we are, our backgrounds, and our education and relate how these experiences shaped our philosophy and the decisions we have made. During the sections on self-reflection, we deviate from the American Psychological Association Style Manual by using our first names and speak from a personal perspective. We believe this provides the readers a more intimate connection with the editors of this book and is more in keeping with the language of self-reflection.

Use of Self

We learned throughout this project that we were similar in the way we looked at decision-making. First, we both knew that decision-making required a way of looking at the world that was synchronous with what we believed about nursing. We both shared a holistic view that nurses, especially public health nurses who we both were, typically hold. For us, this meant that there was no one approach to use when making decisions. We both recognized that decision-making is a fluid process in which self-reflection, listening to others, knowledge of various frameworks, and ways of knowing (Carper, 1992) unfold simultaneously in synergistic process that supports decision-making.

The way we make decisions is influenced by many intra- and interpersonal characteristics like our style, our culture, where we grew up, our education, our personality, and how we perceive the world. We both selected research methods that allowed for our world view or perspective to come through. For example, Marie's hermeneutical study, *The Unfolding Meaning of the Wisdom Experience*, explores the phenomena of wisdom as it unfolds within the context of a nurse-patient relationship and the decision-making process that lies inherent in that experience (Truglio-Londrigan, 2002). The process that Marie uses for decision-making somewhat mirrors the process she used in the hermeneutical method. Gadamer's (1976) philosophical hermeneutical approach is based on the language of conversation and that this conversation provides a medium for understanding as individuals use language to express themselves and listen. This holds true with the decision-making process. Once conversation facilitates understanding via language and listening, not only is understanding the outcome but it is also the ability to identify a decision and act on that decision. This dialogue, questioning, and conversation stand at the center of Gadamer's philosophic hermeneutics (Bernstein, 1983) and portrays an interplay. This interplay is that same looking inward and outward and back inward again earlier described.

Sandy's world view is colored by the research that she does in nursing history. The antecedents to events, knowledge, therapeutic interventions, and the like all contribute to how she approaches decision-making. To her, decisions require an understanding of the historical antecedents. Historiography offers critique of an assortment of historical events, people, issues, therapeutic events, and the like, which offers insight into decision-making. For example, in a 2007 *New York Times* article, McNeil recommended federal guidelines to deal with a severe flu outbreak that were "partly based on a recent study of how 44 cities fared in the 1918 epidemic conducted jointly by the disease centers and the University of Michigan's medical school" (p. A14). In this study, it was the historians and epidemiologists who examined how cities managed during the 1918 flu pandemic. The past provided a way to analyze the possible ways of addressing a potential influenza epidemic today.

Know Yourself

How did we arrive at this juncture? How did we come to be here and think this way? In the following sections of this chapter, we will describe through our own self-reflective process how our philosophical beliefs about decision-making came to be, as well as our own comfort level with choosing a decision, and accepting the risk involved in decision-making. When we make decisions, we each draw from our intra- and interperceptual experiences; however, without self-reflection and awareness of what the self brings to the decision-making process, decisions risk inadequacy or failure.

Marie's Self Reflection

I grew up in "the" Bronx, one of the five boroughs of New York City. No better place in the world, for in the Bronx I was introduced to life, in all its glory and sadness. My parents were high school graduates who worked hard day to day. My mother was a homemaker, my father a postal worker. Both parents were of Italian descent although my father insisted that he was Sicilian; that was somehow different. My maternal grandmother and grandfather lived in the same apartment building as we did. My grandmother was 4 feet, 11 inches tall and packed a punch. My grandfather was 6 feet tall and an alcoholic. They were an integral part of our lives and were involved in my upbringing.

I was baptized Marie Truglio and welcomed into the Catholic church; although as it turns out, I am much more of a spiritual being rather than a religious being. Life has always been one big question to me due to the various experiences I have been introduced to throughout my life.

When I was 3 years old, my sister was born. I remember sitting at my great aunt's kitchen table eating her wonderful pound cake in Queens, New York (another one of the five boroughs) when there was a phone call. I remember that I did not know what they were saying only that all of a sudden the atmosphere in the room changed. My great aunt looked at my father and said "Ann went into labor" to which my father responded, "How can that be? She is not at her due date." This single moment in time changed my life forever. My sister was born with a diagnosis of Down's syndrome. Everyone was so sad and yet I remember I could not understand why. She looked "okay" to me. It is true she did not do much but is that not what all babies do, nothing? When I asked my parents why, they both said that my sister was sick. Sick? She did not appear sick. There never appeared to be any answers to those questions, but I have to say these life experiences created a context for me as being the "searcher": to raise questions and attempt to find answers—even if those answers were "correct" for only a moment in time.

I always asked questions. In the 1960s when riots were on the television every night, others would shake their heads and say "throw them all in jail," while I would question "What is the reason for this?" "Why are these riots taking place?" "What can be done?" Similarly, when the news would account for the number of soldiers who died in Vietnam that day, again I would question, "Is this necessary?" "Who is right?" "What is the truth?" "Is there any truth at all?" My parents would listen to me rant on and on and never tell me to be quiet. They would just listen. This I believe was important. I always knew that I could say and do anything—within reason, of course—and I knew that I always would have my place in this family. I trusted, and this is the trust that is essential to make decisions.

I wanted to be a nurse because I thought I could help; help by stopping the riots, help by stopping the Vietnam War, or help by making my parents proud of something or someone. In any event I made the decision that nursing was going to be my professional commitment. We spoke about risk taking and the choices that we make in decision-making. Well, here was one. I was the first generation in my family to enter in college in the United States. My grandmother had been a teacher in Italy but when she came to this country, she was told that she would never be a teacher here. She was not able to make a decision, the decision was made for her. I was frightened because I could not fail; therefore, I would not fail. I remembered looking at my grandmother and thinking that I was an extension of her. I had to do this. Four years later, I graduated.

Since that time I have embarked on many decisions—some good and some not so good, like the white Volvo my husband and I bought from a car dump in New Jersey. Go figure! I can safely say that we did not use any type of evidence in this move and it was a big risk and a big mistake, one we both learned from. I might add this too is important in decision-making: the importance of self-reflecting and learning from the outcomes of every decision no matter what they are. Nevertheless, other decisions were marked by successes; the decision to marry the man who continues as my husband, the decision to return to school for my masters degree, the decision to build our life and to include children within that life, and finally, the decision to engage in doctoral studies. Every decision portrayed a risk but as I stated earlier, I trusted and this was the trust that my parents modeled for me. They would love me no matter what I said or what I did.

As I stated before, throughout my life, whenever I had to make a decision, I was a searcher. I first would look inward to see what was there. When I found that what I saw was distorted or unclear, I would look outward. Where could I go to find the answers that would clear up this distortion? Once I found what I thought I needed, I would take that knowledge and return to my inner self to see if the distortion was still present or if the picture was clear. What I learned is that for any decision, the comfort of coming to a decision was always short lived. It only lasts for a moment in time because every moment brings newness—hence, my love for hermeneutics as well as the way I conduct myself and look at the world, one moment at a time.

Sandy's Self-Reflection

I was born in 1949 and like Marie, I too was born in the Bronx. I was the second of three daughters and one son. My parents also grew up in the Bronx, attended the same synagogue, and attended the same university in New York City.

My family was not the typical Jewish family. We were Reform Jews, with the roots of this progressive movement stemming back three generations to Germany. We did not grow up in a Jewish neighborhood because my parents wanted us to experience people from all different backgrounds. We lived in a multiethnic and multiracial community that was situated in the northeast section of the Bronx called Wakefield. There were homemade raviolis, a German butcher and deli, a kosher deli, a bakery from Hungarian immigrants, and assorted other ethnic-type food stores that lined the streets under the subway's elevated or "El" pillars (as they were called) on White Plains Road.

My family did things that many of my friends on the block or in most other Bronx neighborhoods did not do. Every summer my parents packed the car, gave each one of us a cardboard box to hold our belongings, and off we went on a camping trip. We were often labeled "gypsies" by friends and family alike because for most of the summer we lived in a tent. My parents started their own hand-guided quilting business, even without having much knowledge about this type of business, and were deeply involved with local Bronx politics, so much so, that my father would recruit the whole family (including some of my dates) to hang the candidates' posters on the subway elevator track poles that lined the avenue near our home.

Both sets of grandparents were born in the United States, which was unusual at the time, at least in our neighborhood. My father's parents died before I was born, so I never met them, but I heard about them, especially about how my grandmother, Lillian Nibur, was a teacher and a suffragist. My mother's grandparents, Monroe and Jennie, both born in the United States but never completed high school, always valued education. It was no surprise to me growing up that I was going to go to college. We saw Monroe and Jennie every Saturday and they played a prominent role in our family's day-to-day life.

When I was 12, my younger sister, who was 7 at the time, died of cystic fibrosis. Given that period of time, little was known about this disease. The cost of care was too high for our family so my father had to find a job in New York City that afforded us health insurance and access to care. He also drove a cab at night to "make ends meet," as my mother would often say. From my memory, we were one of the first families to enroll in the newly formed Health Insurance Plan (HIP) at Montefiore Hospital in the Bronx in about 1962. I remember hearing how the doctors and nurses were trying new treatments for this disease and my sister was given antibiotics, cupping, and other exercises to help her breathe better. In the summer after my sister died, we left for a camping trip across the United States. No matter what had happened that previous year, we kept exploring new environments, new places, and new ideas. One of my father's favorite expressions was "to try it."

Growing up, I loved music, color, dance, and anything that allowed me to move. Today, I probably would be labeled a "kinetic" learner, but in the 1950s and 1960s, learning was mostly done sitting down. My decision to become a nurse probably stemmed from the experience I had with my sister growing up and my need to move. When I decided to become a nurse, my parents were not happy with that decision and tried to steer me toward teaching. They felt nursing was not the right profession to be in, whether because of the images they held about the profession (and that was never clear to me), or that they felt teaching was easier for women who wanted a family. In any event, they agreed with my decision to become a nurse but with the caveat that I attend a collegiate program, not a diploma school. Education was important in my family, and thus shaped my decision about becoming a baccalaureate-prepared nurse.

I met my husband while in nursing school. He attended the dental school a few blocks away. We both marched during the 1960s and early 1970s protest against the Vietnam War, served as health workers at some of the stations that were set up around the city to assist the marchers, and shared many of the same hopes for a country that was undergoing change in civil rights, women's rights, and health care reforms. My husband was born in Rosenheim, Germany, following World War II. I include this piece of history because our two families, both Jewish, both in a health care profession, were so diverse in our cultural backgrounds that decisions we made as a family required real consensus building and an understanding of cultural backgrounds.

My love of history stemmed from my need to understand and explain the world. Growing up, I needed to know. I did not understand the reasons for so many things and always sought answers. My older sister was labeled the "smart one"; my brother was the "man-child"; my sister who died held a special place in the family system because of her illness; I was the middle one and took up the mantle of being the "clown." I could imitate any one of my many teachers, tell jokes, and generally entertained my family on a nightly basis. The humor was my way of knowing and explaining the world.

I did not become interested in nursing history until I returned to school for a master's degree over 10 years following my graduation from my baccalaureate program. It was not until my doctoral work that I learned to use historiography as a research method. It was by raising questions and being ready to explore the historical data to find answers that helped me make the decision to study nursing history. Historical research helped me understand the things that I could no longer laugh about, like why nurses were not valued (perhaps a remnant of the way my family responded to my being a nurse), or why we do not remember nursing's political activity . . . or were they even political or ever involved. (I always remembered the noted public health nurse Lillian Wald and related her to the progressive movement, but somehow that knowledge was not included in my daughter's social study text book that described Wald as a social worker.)

Understanding my background helps me to understand why I made certain decisions about my education, my practice, my research, and my professional goals. It continues to influence me as I make other decisions in life. There are many choices—and many risks. How and what we chose is indicative of our ability to be self-reflective to understand and generate knowledge. How we as nursing professionals help others make decisions also is influenced by both our backgrounds. Being self-reflective and understanding who we are is essential to the decision-making process.

Self-Reflection Assists Decision-Making

Both of us were born in the Bronx in New York City and are both part of the "baby boomer" population that exploded following World War II. Both of our fathers served in World War II. Both had sisters who had health-related issues that left indelible marks. We both grew up in family systems where grandparents were involved and education was important. Our educational experiences were different because Marie went to Catholic school and Sandy went to Bronx public schools. In terms of religion, Marie would classify her family deeply rooted in the practice of Catholicism while Sandy's family espoused the more liberal attitudes of Reform Judaism. We each chose a 4-year baccalaureate degree in nursing because college education was highly valued in our families. Even our choice of clinical setting, public health nursing, was similar because Sandy enjoyed being outside and moving, and Marie felt there was a potential to make an impact for the greater good. Both agree that there was greater autonomy and freedom to choose in this setting than in others. Serendipity brought us together to work at the same institution, teach the same course, and write this book, but it was also our backgrounds and the knowledge we gained from being self-reflective that led us to this point as well.

The decisions we make and the ones we assist others make in our practice all have some elements of our past interacting with the decision, whether consciously or unconsciously. This then makes it so imperative for all of us who are in health care professions to be aware of what we consider worthwhile, such as a special treatment, the health care provider we visit, the hospital we select, or the treatment plan we follow. Do we exercise to stay healthy or avoid any kind of health-promoting or preventative-type activities? Do we smoke or do we have difficulty watching anyone who does? What are our values related to health care, and how do our biases affect the very people we are caring for? The practice of self-reflection, then, becomes essential to any decisions that nurses make.

Conclusion

In this first chapter, we wanted to introduce ourselves and through self-reflection demonstrate how past life experience does in fact affect how we live in the world, how we perceive the world, and how we conduct ourselves when making decisions. To us, decision-making is more than a model or framework, it is a philosophy intimately intertwined with our view of the world. Self-reflection creates awareness and knowledge building. It also helped us formulate our philosophy about decision-making. Our histories share many similarities and differences, and the decisions we make and assist others make reflect this.

We wanted to write Chapter 1 because it became clear to us that how we engage in the decision-making process has more to do with philosophy than any one approach to decision-making. This philosophy has unfolded over the years as a result of life experiences. Self-reflection allows one access to this knowledge and gives a clearer picture of ourselves, so that we can ultimately use this knowledge when we make decisions and help the various constituents in our practice make their decisions. Self-reflection serves as an integral part for all nurses engaging in decision-making process. An awareness of who we are opens us up to the possibility of who others may be and how we interact with them in therapeutic relationships. Reflective decision-making requires self-reflection when using the variety of thoughtful approaches we present in this text and beyond.

References

Bernstein, R. (1983). *Beyond objectivism and relativism: Science, hermeneutics, and praxis.* Philadelphia: University of Pennsylvania Press.

Buchanan, L., & O'Connell, A. (2006). A brief history of decision-making. *Harvard Business Review, 84*(1), 32–37.

Carper, B. A. (1992). Philosophical inquiry in nursing: An application. In J. E. Kikuchi & H. Simmons (Eds.). *Philosophical inquiry in nursing* (pp. 71–80). London: Sage Publications.

Gadamer, H. G. (1976). *Philosophical hermeneutics* (D. Ling, Trans. & Ed.). Los Angeles, CA: University of California Press.

McNeil, D. G. (2007, February 7). Closings and cancellations top advice on flu outbreak. *The New York Times,* A14.

Mountford, B., & Rogers, L. (1996). Using individual and group reflection in and on assessment as a tool for effective learning. *Journal of Advanced Nursing, 24,* 1127–1134.

O'Donnell, J. P., Lewenson, S. B., & Keith-Anderson, K. (2000). Who am I?: Teaching nurse practitioner students to develop self-reflective practice. In M. Katherine Crabtree (Ed.). *Teaching clinical decision-making in advanced nursing practice.* Washington, DC: National Organization of Nurse Practitioner Faculties.

Truglio-Londrigan, M. (2002). An analysis of wisdom: An experience in nursing practice. *The Journal of the New York State Nurses Association, 33* (2), 24–30.

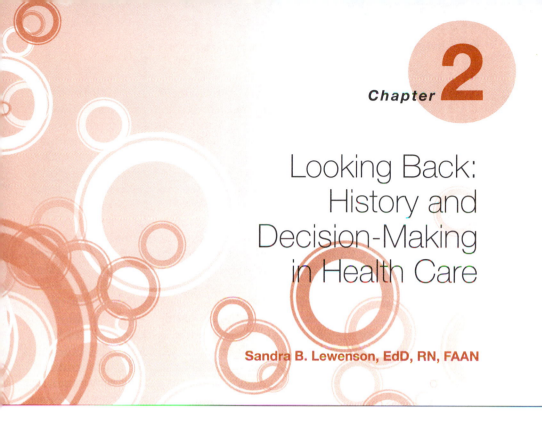

Chapter 2

Looking Back: History and Decision-Making in Health Care

Sandra B. Lewenson, EdD, RN, FAAN

Nurses make decisions every day that affect the health of the individuals, families, and communities they serve. They make decisions about the use of clinical interventions, the use of their political vote, the education of nurses, the application of new technologies, and a myriad of others as well—yet when nurses make decisions, they often use decision-making frameworks that do not take into account past practices. Nelson and Gordon (2004) write about the "rhetoric of rupture," stating that nurses often discard and distance themselves from their past, leaving huge gaps in their knowledge. Nurses continually reinvent themselves and their practice at the expense of their history. Without understanding and valuing past contributions to practice or to society, nurses contribute to the "nursism" or bias toward the caring role that pervades this society (Lewenson, 1993). The omission of what nurses do on a day-to-day basis is lost to both current and future generations of nurses and to others who might benefit from such knowledge.

In 1939, nurse historian Mary Roberts wrote that "trends and events of today are the results of past experience as well as of varying conceptions of both present and future needs" (p. 1). Roberts recognized the need to examine the history of nursing to see how the profession could move forward. Another nurse historian Teresa Christy (1978) explained how she could not "emphasize enough the relevance of an understanding of yesterday's problems for illumination of today's issues and concomitant potential for tomorrow's solutions" (p. 5).Whether nurses choose to use history in their decision-making process, history impacts their decisions. Thus, as part of a reflective decision-making process, nurses need to know their history to make meaningful decisions about their current and future work. This chapter explores why history helps nurses in their decision-making process as well as briefly describes the history of decision-making in nursing.

Historiography provides a way of understanding the past and therefore provides a framework in which to study and apply history to decision-making. Although it is beyond the scope of this chapter to discuss the steps used in historiography, it identifies some of the historical studies that contribute to the evidence used in practice and professional growth. The case study opening this chapter illustrates how graduate nursing students use historical evidence to support the decision-making process in a community health clinical experience. The historiographies presented in this chapter offer examples of how history informs the decision-making efforts of nurses. The case study closing this chapter provides an illustration of how historical knowledge about nursing roles would help current nurses in their practice.

Case Study

A Community Assessment of the Lower East Side of New York City, 1893

What began as a study to look at the Lower East Side of New York City as Lillian Wald may have seen it when she established the Henry Street Settlement became an exciting exercise for students to explore how decisions were made. Nurses need to be able to assess a community and determine the types of services that would most benefit the community. To teach nurses how to assess a community, prioritize primary health care needs of the community, plan and develop an appropriate intervention, and examine the impact of their decisions, a look at historical data was used. In this case study, graduate nursing students interested in community and the Henry Street Settlement in the Lower East Side of New York City joined in doing a historical community assessment as part of their requirement for a master's project. To complete this requirement, they examined the period of time in which the Henry Street Settlement house was first organized.

The Henry Street Settlement was started in 1893 by two public health nurses, Lillian Wald and her friend, Mary Brewster. Using the demographic data, photographs, and selected writings from 1893 enabled the current students to more fully understand what Wald and Brewster might have seen when they first established the nurses' settlement house on the Lower East Side of New York. The study helped students learn why Wald and Brewster opened a nurses' settlement house in the area, the kinds of health care issues that they found, and the impact that their nursing decisions had on the health of that community. In addition, this project enabled students to look at the professional and health care issues over time and see how they compared with those of today. They used history to help them understand the role of the visiting nurse, the political activism that the nurses exhibited, and the obligation to society that nurses continue to maintain now in the twenty-first century. They also used their findings to help them in making decisions about community health initiatives in the same community over 100 years later.

Students studied the Lower East Side community, specifically the area designated as the 7th and 10th Ward. In the late nineteenth century, New York City was divided into wards rather than the present-day census tracts, and data was therefore collected according to ward and sanitary districts. The students examined the demographics; morbidity and mortality rates; immigration patterns; police, fire, and sanitation support services; educational, religious, and social institutions in the community; and the political and nursing issues of that period. Students identified the priority needs in the community and compared their ideas with the actual contributions of the nurses at Henry Street. The students learned about the overcrowded living conditions that so many of the immigrants who populated the Lower East Side found in the tenements. In 1893 the total population in Manhattan (a borough of New York City in which the Lower East Side was a small section) totaled 1,758,000. About 1,332,773 or 69 percent of the total population, however, lived in the tenements of the Lower East Side. There were 180,359 children under the age of 5 (*Annual Report*, 1909).

The data showed that the residents of the Lower East Side came from Italy, Germany, Hungary, Russia, and other European countries. Once they arrived in the United States and moved to the Lower East Side, they found the tenements waiting for them. They experienced six-floor walk-up apartments, a lack of running water (this was prior to the cold-water flats that evolved following the inclusion of sinks in the tenements), outdoor plumbing until plumbing moved onto the hallway of each floor, as well as poor ventilation and poor lighting. Families, regardless of their size, resided in the two rooms that made up the apartments of the early tenements. Lack of privacy was just one of the many insults to the human condition that existed for those who lived in the tenements. The Tenement Museum in New York shows what life in the tenements was like and students were able to access the Web site (www.tenement.org) as well as personally visit this setting.

The inadequate housing conditions as well as the inhumane work conditions of so many of the immigrants contributed to the poor health conditions that they experienced. Some of the findings showed that infants accounted for 25 percent of all deaths in the community and that children under 5 accounted for 40 percent of all deaths in the community. The top causes of death in 1893 were pneumonia, phthis (pulmonary tuberculosis), digestive organ diseases, heart disease, and diphtheria. Infectious diseases made up 42 percent of the deaths in this community, with pneumonia, phthis, diarrhea, and diphtheria leading the list of these illnesses (*Annual Report*, 1909; *Annual Report*, 1897).

Students learned that between 1892 and 1893 there was a 30 percent increase in suicide and that immigrants accounted for 80 percent of these suicides. They further examined how the social, economic, and political factors around 1893 may have affected the suicide rates among the immigrant population. The financial depression of 1893 in the United States surely may have contributed to the increase in the number of suicides during this period. Students explored crime statistics, literacy rates, and houses of worship, social services, and other important community support. They could visualize the effects of—or lack of—these supports by the outcomes they observed in the morbidity and mortality rates (*Annual Report*, 1897).

Students also read some of Wald's writings and began to learn about the programs that Wald and Brewster, along with the Henry Street nurses, brought to the community. The Henry Street visiting nurses, the students learned, lived at the settlement house and became neighbors of the families they served. They read about Wald's famous "baptism by fire" where she meets a young child who led her through the streets of the Lower East Side to visit her mother who had been hemorrhaging for 2 days in bed after a difficult childbirth. Wald's graphic description provides a stark reality that students could relate to the experience. Wald wrote (1915):

> Through Hester and Division streets we went to the end of Ludlow; past odorous fish-stands, for the streets were a market-place, unregulated, unsupervised, unclean; past evil-smelling, uncovered garbage-cans; and—perhaps worst of all, where so many little children played. . . . The child led me on through a tenement hallway, across a court where open and unscreened closets were promiscuously used by men and women, up into a rear tenement, by slimy steps whose accumulated dirt was augmented that day by the mud of the streets, and finally into the sickroom. . . . Although the family of seven shared their two rooms with boarders . . . and although

the sick woman lay on a wretched, unclean bed, soiled with a hemorrhage two days old, they were not degraded human beings . . . that morning's experience was a baptism of fire." (pp. 5–6)

Soon after Wald met the family of seven, she and her friend, Mary Brewster, began the Henry Street Settlement for the expressed purpose of improving the unhealthy living conditions they found in the community. Both nurses were social activists and strove to improve the life of the residents of the Lower East Side through political action and nursing interventions. Wald, especially, felt that nurses had the knowledge and skills to advocate political changes to improve the health of the families in the community. Wald (1900/1991) explained that

among the many opportunities for civic and altruistic work pressing on all sides nurses having superior advantages in their practical training should not rest content with being only nurses, but should use their talents wherever possible in reform and civic movements. (p. 318)

Wald's belief that nurses were poised to advocate for change in the social, economic, and political conditions of the community in which they lived, led to many of the reforms that contributed to the health of the citizens in the community. For example, Wald visited families in their home providing access to nursing care; organized well-baby classes for new mothers; advocated the first school nurse program in New York City which placed a nurse in a city school; established a playground in the community, one of the first of its kind; and fostered an intellectual community of nurses who actively lobbied for social and political changes that supported the health of the citizens in the community.

Given the data that the students collected in their community assessment, they felt that there was synergy between the programs that Wald established and the data they collected. Through the data, they witnessed the sights that Wald and Brewster saw as they made decisions to provide primary health care in the community. Students also saw the similarities between 1893 and the current period of time. What seemed to exist in 1893 continued to exist in a different (but similar) form. Access to care, a rise in tuberculosis, women as primary caregivers, a close relationship between poverty and access to care, large groups of immigrant populations, the need for social and political activism to support health care initiatives, and environmental factors affecting the health of children and adults in the community continue to be concerns in the same community in the twenty-first century. While variations exist today on the particular environmental concerns, patterns of immigration, and political climate, what continues to be a constant is the need for nurses to make decisions about care and provide leadership in improving the health of individuals, families, and the communities they serve.

The graduate students' use of history to learn about community assessments, community action, and nursing's role in political activism helped decide the kinds of health-promoting interventions they could use in their own community clinical experience. Understanding the history of Henry Street offers a way for students to see how decisions were made in the past and to value the remarkable outcomes that these decisions rendered in the nursing profession and the health of the community. They used some of the ideas of the past and introduced them with the ideas that they learned about primary health care in the twenty-first century. Teaching parenting skills, like Wald did in 1893, were one of the projects students initiated at Henry Street's abused women's shelter. Classes in parenting, nutrition, and other health promotion–type activities, which reflected current thinking of the nursing students, continued in the kinds of programming that the original public health nurses of the settlement house offered to the community. Students also saw the leadership displayed by Wald and other public health nurses in the late nineteenth and early twentieth centuries and how their activism continued to be a model for them today.

Nursing History Informs the Decision-Making Process

History provides a knowledge base that allows nurses to better understand their practice and profession. Knowing the evolution of nursing care, or the reasons why nurses for almost 100 years debate the educational level into practice, or why each state requires separate licensing of nursing professionals, affords nurses a way to understand the challenges that the profession has faced over time. Historical understanding allows for thoughtful decisions that facilitate innovation and change. Sometimes, however, tradition is mistaken for historical knowledge and thus, confounds the decision-making process. Pape (2003) states that an organization's valuing of tradition may cause an organization to oppose changes in practice (p. 156). While tradition is part of history, understanding the origins of tradition through historical research allows a basis for comparison, critique, and ultimately decisions that allow for change. Historical research rather than tradition should be the key element used in providing evidence to support decision-making efforts of nursing professionals.

Historical evidence provides depth and context to issues nurses face today and as a result, the American Association for the History of Nursing (AAHN) supports the inclusion of nursing history in the curriculum. Keeling (2001) writes in an AAHN position paper, that "nurses in the 21st century will need more than sheer information; they will need a greater sensitivity to contextual variables and ambiguity if they are to critically evaluate the information they receive" (Keeling, 2001). Nurses need the ability to study, understand, and value history. Integrating nursing history into nursing curricula at all levels is essential to help nurses identify their history; obtain the necessary skills to explore, study, and understand their history; and to ultimately use history in their decision-making process (Lewenson, 2004; Keeling, 2001).

Studying history provides nurses a conceptualization of the modern nursing movement from 1873 to the present day and affords a continuity between the past and present. This continuity allows for nurses to avoid the familiar adage: "Those who do not study history are doomed to repeat it." For nurses, not using history in the decision-making process may waste valuable time and resources in reinventing what was already previously discovered to work (or not work). Not using history also may deny the success of decisions made in nursing education, practice, research, or administration. Nurses need to know what worked and what did not work, and how they can seek the data to support decisions that need to be made by nurses. History is a valuable resource as a knowledge base and allows for its use as a form of evidence. The graduate students in the case study "saw" the conditions the newly immigrated families experienced in 1893 and some of the primary health care needs that Wald and her colleagues at the Henry Street Settlement met. Without understanding the historical significance of the Lower East Side, the graduate students would miss the origins of some of the socially minded programs and ideology of the settlement houses that continue to exist in this area today.

Strumpf and Tomes (1993) examined the historical use of restraints in "troublesome patients" in the United States during the nineteenth century. They observed a difference between the common use of restraints in the United States versus the infrequent use of such devices in Great Britain. The cultural beliefs about the kind of care that these patients, including the mentally ill and the elderly, differed historically in both countries and the outcomes of care varied as well. Strumpf and Tomes recognized the need to study history in order for nurse administrators and nurses to examine their decisions about the use of restraints and to give them a better understanding of why they continue to use them with the elderly when evidence does not support the use of these devices.

> Contemporary observers often assume that this modern restraint crisis is a peculiar product of the late twentieth century, with its large population of aged and chronically ill, fiscal crisis, institutional overcrowding, and staff turnover. . . . Many of the contemporary dilemmas involving physical restraint can be traced back to an earlier "restraint crisis" that occurred during the middle of the nineteenth century. (Strumpf & Tomes, 1993, p. 4)

Like Strumpf and Tomes, historians search for reasons why things occurred and do so in the hope of informing contemporary issues that need thoughtful decisions. When nurses do a nursing assessment on a patient, they start with a nursing history. Nurses would not be able to appropriately assess their patients or develop plans of action without one. If that is the case, why would nursing leaders, educators, practitioners, researchers, and the like attempt to make decisions without getting the history first?

A Historical Look at Decision-Making in Nursing

In exploring the use of nursing history in decision-making, it would be important to look at the history of decision-making in nursing or when and how nurses made decisions. Questions arise such as whether nurses actually made decisions overtly or did they "downplay" their own reasoning abilities to avoid alienating physicians if they assumed a more autonomous role? Did nurses always make decisions about care and about the profession? If so, what kinds of evidence did they use to make these decisions? How did they document these decisions? Were nurses more autonomous in their roles as nurses, such as the ones that Hallett, Abendstern, and Wade (2006) or that Keeling (2006) describe in their work or were nurses merely following physician orders as they cared for their patients? How did nursing's close ties with the women's movement in the late 1800s and early 1900s affect the way nurses made decisions? Were nurses afraid of alienating politicians who could possibly assist the nursing profession obtain nursing registration laws as Lewenson (1993) suggests or did they speak out in favor of women suffrage, regardless of how it affected these politicians? Did Wald and Brewster use the same available demographic data as in the case study about the Lower East Side when determining the need for health care programs in the community? Have nurses historically used "evidence" to support their practice? If so, what kind of evidence did they use and how did they find the evidence?

Nursing research, important to the decision-making process, evolved in the profession as nursing educators and leaders called for nurses to base their clinical decisions on empirical evidence. Nursing educator R. Louise McManus (1961) asked the question: "What is the place of nursing research—yesterday, today, and tomorrow" (p. 76) and examined the evolution of nursing research. She understood the need to look at how research influenced the decisions of nursing leaders in order to plan for the future in nursing. McManus explained that nursing research—or the "methodological search for nursing knowledge"—differed from other professional groups because early studies focused more on nursing education and service rather than on practice.

She reasoned that interest in nursing research differed from other professions because of the different "pressures upon the profession as a whole by social, political, and economic forces and the impact on nursing advances in scientific knowledge" (p. 76).

McManus (1961) highlights the early research efforts of Nightingale, and the later studies of M. Adelaide Nutting, Isabel Stewart, and others who examined nursing education and the status of the profession. The studies, McManus said, usually were implemented by the professional organizations, like the American Society of Superintendents of Training Schools for Nurses (which was renamed the National League of Nursing Education in 1912, and then the National League for Nursing in 1952), and as a result focused more on the issues related to education. Nurse educators, like Stewart, valued research and participated in and led many such endeavors such as her noted time-and-motion studies. Another noted nursing leader, Virginia Henderson, published early scientific studies such as the one McManus includes on "Medical and Surgical Asepsis" in 1939. Structure studies of how the professional organizations should look also were done and dramatically influenced the change in nursing organizations in the early 1950s.

McManus's (1961) examination of history provides a view of the development of nursing research prior to the early 1960s that explains as well as raises questions about nursing's interest in research and the subsequent culture of research. She noted that the way nursing organized around issues of practice and service as well as one of the first graduate educational programs for nurses situated in Teachers College, Columbia University (a college for teachers), was indicative of the kinds of studies and research of early nursing. McManus (1961) wrote that: "This happenstance of teachers pushing toward education and toward a teacher training institution for the first graduate programs may well have affected the course of nursing's development considerably" (p. 79).

Many in nursing were interested in knowledge building to support decisions in nursing. In her 1934 article in the *American Journal of Nursing*, Sister M. Bernice Beck called for nurses to base their practice on scientific principles rather than on outdated models that supported a paternalistic hierarchy. Nurses, especially educators and administrators, needed to have a "scientific attitude," which Beck described as being

> . . . openminded, ready to learn the truth and accept it; observant, keen, clear-minded, cautious, alert, vigorous, original, and independent in thinking; she carefully weighs all the evidence and overlooks no factor which may influence the results; allows no personal preferences to influence decisions; holds only tentative scientific convictions, because aware that we have not yet arrived at the end of knowledge, but are constantly wresting more secrets from the hidden depths of Nature." (p. 580)

The early move toward basing practice on nursing research required that nurses examine the way they carried out procedures and not just accept what they did without first examining the outcomes of their actions. Beck wrote that the teacher of nursing arts

> never insists that procedures, as taught, are the last word; that the unfounded statements of textbooks must be accepted without question, and that the ordering physician must be looked upon as an infallible authority. On the contrary, she urges her students to find out why things are done as they are; whether there are not better ways of doing them; to challenge statements, to ask for proofs, to think for themselves, to make individual contributions. (p. 581)

Students were expected to learn to question and to make decisions based on the response to their questions. Decisions were not to be made by rote; rather they needed to be made using research data. Harmer and Henderson (1940) in their noted text, *The Principles and Practice of Nursing*, included a section on the "Professional Responsibilities in Relation to Method." Nurses were to "accept the responsibility for studying its procedures and designing its method" (p. 469).

In order to understand how decisions in nursing are made and the kinds of decision-making models or frameworks available, it is important to remember to place decisions within a context that looks at the particular period in which those decisions are made. The students in the case study presented earlier in this chapter examined the demographic data and the morbidity and mortality rates of the Lower East Side within the context of the late nineteenth-century United States. They explored the meaning of immigration within the social, political, and economic period of the day. In this way, they could compare and contrast the health care decisions that were made by nurses during that period with the more contemporary decisions made today in the same community. This may be beyond the scope of this chapter, but it is something to consider when looking at history and decision-making in nursing.

Historical Critiques Assist Decision-Making in Nursing

Historiography provides the data and the necessary critique that nurses require in their decision-making process. Lewenson (2007) shows how studies in nursing education, practice, and administration provide historical evidence that nurses may use when making decisions on such issues as appropriate educational levels in nursing, the role of the nurse practitioner, and resolving the nursing shortage. Studies like the one that Whelan (2005) did on exploring the demise of private duty nursing in the United States provides data for a discussion about nursing short-age, staffing issues, and changes in the hospital settings. R. A. Seeger Jablonski's (2003) study examines the history of the nurse practitioner movement and the effect on nursing education at the Virginia Commonwealth University (VCU). The historical account at VCU serves as a way of knowing what happened to this particular program and serves as an example of how other programs may have fared during the same time period.

Historical studies provide explanations, connections, and relation-ships among variables in the past and can be used to assist today's nurses in the decision-making process. For example, understanding the history of nursing's clinical practice provides knowledge of what worked in the past and perhaps how it can improve. Historical studies, such as Keeling's (2006) "Medicines in the Work of Henry Street Settlement Visiting Nurses," explores the role the settlement nurses played in giv-ing medications and nursing interventions, thus, illuminating ques-tions about the work of visiting nurses, autonomy, prescriptive privileges, and legal boundaries of practice today. These visiting nurses in the late nineteenth and early twentieth century gave medications that were sometimes prescribed, as well as gave medications that were not. These nurses sought the over-the-counter treatments that both nurses and laypeople often used to heal a wound or cure a cold.

Keeling describes how these treatments fell somewhere in the mid-dle, using Lavinia Dock's (author of the 1898 *Materia Medica for Nurses*) term describing the role of the nurse as being in the "middle place" or somewhere between "professional medical service and unskilled fam-ily caregiving" (2006, p. 9). Keeling also noted that nurses did not write about their administration of medications, frequently taking this part of their work for granted as well as trying to minimize it. The research showed how the Henry Street Settlement House (HSS) visiting nurses challenged the boundaries of the early nurse practice acts and sought to provide access to care, often diagnosing, prescribing, and carrying out treatments, without the direct supervision as was required by law of the physician.

Why Keeling's 2006 research is important to decision-making is found in any number of contemporary discussions addressing the role of nurses, autonomy of practice, nurse practitioner licensure, the move toward a doctor of nursing practice, changes in licensure for health care professionals, and other issues affecting nursing education, prac-tice, and research. Keeling uncovers how little is known of the work of the HSS visiting nurses. This group of professionals often has been studied from a social-political perspective about their activities and the effect they had on improving the environment for the families and in-dividuals they served in the Lower East Side community in New York City rather than on their actual clinical practice.

Nurses today who work with families in the home may also struggle with dispensing advice about medications and offering information about health care interventions typically found in the home. Families today have greater access and knowledge about these medications, but may be hampered by restrictions set by nurse practice acts that prohibit nurses prescribing medications. Given the greater access to the Internet, television, newspapers, or magazines, consumer levels of understanding have been raised and with that their expectations about care.

This "middle place" that Dock describes in her 1898 book and Keeling refers to in her 2006 article is specifically directed toward nurses. Dock wrote her book for nurses to learn about drugs and their administration from the standpoint of what nurses needed to know rather than from what physicians needed to know. Until 1890, when Dock first published her book, the medical perspective was the only one available. Nurses learned about pharmacology from the books available at the time, and not until Dock wrote hers specifically for nurses was the nursing intervention and role of the nurse addressed.

Another historical study by Hallett, Abendstern, and Wade (2006) examines the autonomous clinical practice of the industrial nurse in England around the mid-twentieth century. In the cotton factories, concern for the health of the workers, mostly women, was in the hands of the "welfare officer." The welfare officer usually had formal nurse's training or in some instances they were not nurses, but had first-aid training. Hallett, Abendstern, and Wade conclude that little is known about the clinical side of industrial nursing and the history of this specialty has been overlooked in general by nursing. Hallett, Abendstern, and Wade used oral histories of cotton factory workers as well as three of the welfare officers to gain insight into the autonomous nature of this role and how it shaped the care of a group of cotton workers in the middle of the twentieth century. The outcome of the study describes the values that these particular nurses ascribed to in the fulfillment of their responsibilities. The welfare officers who were nurses worked autonomously providing nursing interventions, that like Keeling's study, revealed they dispensed medications and nursing treatments that relied on their own nursing assessment and diagnosis. Hallett, Abendstern, and Wade (2006) stated that these nurses were imbued "with a sense of autonomy and a consciousness of the 'expert' nature of their role. They were not willing to be 'told their job' by mill owners" (p. 103). The interventions were mostly first aid in nature and did not seem to cover preventative, screening-type interventions that would have promoted health care of employees. The written record is more limited and the history of this period is captured mostly through oral history, without which, the knowledge would no longer be accessible (Hallett, Abendstern, & Wade, 2006, p. 103).

Both Keeling (2006) and Hallett, Abendstern, and Wade (2006) provide today's nurses with data of what was done in the past. They uncover the history of working nurses and make connections between then and now. Keeler, for example, links the work of the Henry Street nurses in the early twentieth century and the role of nurse practitioners today. Contemporary nurses struggle with decisions about advanced practice, nurse practice acts, and collaborating partnerships with physicians that would all benefit in the knowledge that these two historiographies presented. Uncovering of the history informs not only the practice, but the education and research as well and thus affects nursing outcomes today and in the future. Today's professionals can learn from the wisdom, knowledge, mistakes, and vision of those earlier nurses.

Another Case Study

In 1996 when I was an instructor in a community health course on the Lower East Side in New York City, one of the students, who was a registered nurse returning to school for a baccalaureate degree in nursing, was visiting a "client" of the Henry Street Settlement Home Health Care agency in the home. The student professionally worked as a cardiac care nurse and was proficient in providing high-level care using the latest technology in cardiac care. However, when she entered this client's home during the community clinical rotation, she said she was shocked at the odor emanating from the client's feet and had difficulty knowing what her responsibilities were in this case. She wanted to know what could be done for this client, because there were no medical orders and she felt she could not do anything without them.

The goal of the community experience at the Henry Street Settlement (where the visiting nursing service had separated from the agency in 1944) was to visit clients who received homemaking services in the home. Students were expected to develop a nursing plan of care after completing a nursing assessment of the client, the client's concerns, the homemaker's concern, and an assessment of the home and community resources. When I visited the client's home with the student nurse and saw the caked-on dirt and smelled the odor from the feet, I asked the homemaker to prepare a basin of warm water so that we could soak the client's feet. We instituted a nursing intervention, bathing of the feet, so that we could further assess the skin color, the temperature, and the integrity of the skin. As we bathed the feet, the student spoke with the client and began to build trust with him and develop a rapport with the homemaker. Following the simple "nursing" procedure, the student patted the feet dry, continued to assess the feet, and began to teach the client about proper foot care.

The student said on the walk back to Henry Street that while she could operate efficiently in the hospital setting, the home-care setting created new challenges to her perceived role of the nurse. She was unaware of what visiting nurses did or had done in the past. She lacked historical perspective that might have assisted her in understanding this middle ground where nurses provide nursing care autonomously. The autonomous role that she was learning in the community clinical experience had ties with earlier nurses in the same community. Yet not knowing the past creates challenges for her and all nurses who make decisions in their practice.

Conclusion

History provides today's nurses with an "overarching conceptual framework that allows us to more fully understand the disparate meaning of nursing and the different experiences of nurses" (D'Antonio, 2003, p.1). Lynaugh and Reverby (1987) said that history "provides us with the tools to examine the full range of human existence and to assess the constraints under which decisions are made" (Lynaugh & Reverby, 1987, p. 4). Without understanding nursing history, decisions are at risk of failing and repeating past errors. Historiography provides a way of knowing and understanding of what has gone on before, what is happening now, and what may be expected in the future. If all knowledge has a historical dimension, then nurses need to take this dimension into account whenever a decision is made. All decisions, regardless of the decision-making approach that nurses may use, also must include an historical dimension in the matrix. Like the case studies presented and the historiographies identified, nurses can learn from understanding the past and using this understanding to support the kinds of decisions that they make today.

> History is alive, and the search for answers in history is useful for solving present difficulties, directing behavior, and accomplishing the objectives of the nursing profession. When the answers are found, it is not the end. It is the beginning (Austin, 1978, p. viii).

References

Annual Report of the Board of Health of the Department of Health of the City of New York VII, 1908. (1909). New York: Martin, Printers, & Stationers.

Annual Report of the Board of Health of the Health Department of the City of New York for the year ending December 31, 1893. (1897). New York: Martin B. Brown, Printers and Stationers.

Austin, A. L. (1978). Foreword. In M. Louise Fitzpatrick, ed. *Historical studies in nursing: Papers presented at the 15th Annual Stewart Conference on Research in Nursing March 1977*, pp. vii–viii. New York: Teachers College Press.

Beck, M. B. (1934). Coordinating the teaching of sciences and nursing practice: Underlying scientific principles in nursing practice. *The American Journal of Nursing*, 34(6), pp. 579–586. Located through JSTOR Wednesday, January 17, 2007 at 10:46:38.

Christy, T. E. (1978). The hope of history. In M. Louise Fitzpatrick, Ed. *Historical studies in nursing: Papers presented at the 15th Annual Stewart Conference on Research in Nursing March 1977* (pp. 3–11). New York: Teachers College Press.

D'Antonio, P. (2003). Editor's note. *Nursing History Review, 11*, p. 1.

Dock, L. L. (1898). *Text-book of materia medica for nurses* (3rd ed. rev. and enlarged). New York: G. P. Putnam's Sons.

Hallett, C., Abendstern, M., & Wade, L. (2006). Industry and autonomy in early occupational health nursing: The welfare officers of the Lancashire cotton mills in the mid-twentieth century. *Nursing History Review, 14*, pp. 89–109.

Harmer, B., & Henderson, V. (1940). *Textbook of the principles and practice of nursing* (4th ed., revised). New York: MacMillan Company.

Keeling, A. (2001). *Nursing history in the curriculum: Preparing nurses for the 21st century*. AAHN position paper. Retrieved August 8, 2006, from http://aahn.org/position.html

Keeling, A. (2006). Medicines in the work of Henry Street Settlement Visiting Nurses. *Nursing History Review, 14*, pp. 7–30. New York: Springer.

Lewenson, S. B. (1993). *Taking charge: Nursing, suffrage, and feminism in America, 1873–1920*. New York: Garland.

Lewenson, S. B. (2004). Integrating nursing history into the curriculum. *Journal of Professional Nursing, 20*(6), 347–380.

Lewenson, S. B. (2007). Chapter 12: Historical research in practice, education, and administration. In H. J. Speziale & D. R. Carpenter (Eds.). *Qualitative research in nursing: Advancing the humanistic imperative*, 4th ed. (pp. 273–300). Philadelphia: Lippincott.

Lynaugh, J., & Reverby, S. (1987). Thoughts on the nature of history. *Nursing Research, 36*(1), 4, 69.

McManus, R. L. (1961). Nursing research—Its evolution. *American Journal of Nursing, 61*(4), pp. 76–79. Retrieved February 26, 2007, from http://links.jstor.org/sici?sici=0002-936X%28196104%2961%3A4%3C76%3ANRIE%3E2.0.CO%3B2-P

Nelson, S., & Gordon, S. (2004). The rhetoric of rupture: Nursing as practice with a history? *Nursing Outlook, 52*, 255–261.

Pape, T. M. (2003). Evidence-based nursing practice: To infinity and beyond. *Journal of Continuing Education in Nursing, 34*(4), 154–161.

Roberts, M. (1939). Current events and trends in nursing. *American Journal of Nursing, 39*(1), 1–8. Retrieved January 17, 2007, from http://links.jstor.org/sici?sici=0002-936X%28193901%2939%3A1%3C1%3ACEATIN%3E2.0.CO%3B2-U

Seeger Jablonski, R. A. (2003). Sparks to wildfires: The emergence and impact of nurse practitioner education at Virginia Commonwealth University 1974–1991. Nursing History Review, 11, 167–185. New York: Springer Publishing Company.

Strumpf, N. E., & Tomes, N. (1993). Restraining the troublesome patient: A historical perspective on a contemporary debate. Nursing History Review, 1, 1–24.

Wald, L. D. (1900). Work of women in municipal affairs. Proceedings of the Sixth Annual Convention of the American Society of Superintendents of Nurses (pp. 54–57). Harrisburg, PA: Harrisburg Pub. Reprinted in Birnbach, N., & Lewenson, S. B. (Eds.) (1991). First words: Selected addresses from the National League for Nursing, 1894–1933 (pp. 315–318). New York: NLN.

Wald, L. D. (1915). The house on Henry Street. New York: Henry Holt and Company.

Whelan, J. (2005). 'A necessity in the nursing world': The Chicago Nurses Professional Registry, 1913–1950. Nursing History Review, 13, 49–75.

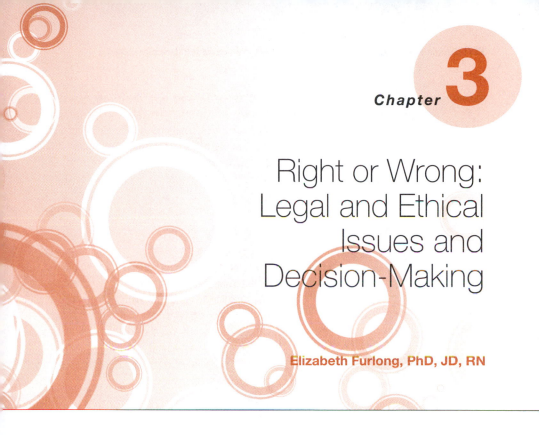

Chapter 3

Right or Wrong: Legal and Ethical Issues and Decision-Making

Elizabeth Furlong, PhD, JD, RN

Nurses make decisions every day that must take into account laws and ethical standards. Therefore, in order to make appropriate decisions, nurses require an understanding of how laws, ethics, and nursing interface. This chapter provides a compelling case study that occurred in Nebraska and underscores the importance of nurses being constantly aware of changing laws, petition drives, and ballot initiatives. The Nebraska case study, as this case will be called throughout the chapter, shows how legal and ethical factors affect clinical nursing practice and how nurses must consider both aspects when making decisions in their practice.

Nebraska Case Study

In the summer and fall of 2006, a group of individuals from states outside of Nebraska wrote and financially funded a petition drive to obtain enough signatures to promote an amendment to the Nebraska state constitution (Stoddard, 2006). The proposed amendment was titled "Nebraskans for a Humane Care Amendment." For the proponents, it would ensure a legal mandate that all individuals in Nebraska would not have medical interventions nor food and water withheld nor withdrawn in terminal conditions. The amendment included a statement that the proposed amendment would respect advance directives of individuals who had fully expressed language in their advance directive about the withholding of food and water in terminal conditions. The opponents of this petition had the following concerns:

1. The initiative was from out-of-state.
2. There was only one or two Nebraskans who had any involvement—which was a minimal legalistic engagement.
3. If passed, the policy would create ethical dilemmas for patients, family members, and health care providers because the proposed amendment mandate did not reflect medical nor ethical best practices for patients in terminal conditions.
4. The amendment would take decision-making away from parents about their children's conditions.

In early September 2006, the Nebraska secretary of state ruled that the petition organizers had not obtained enough valid signatures to have the petition put on the November 2006 election ballot (Stoddard, 2006). He disqualified many of the signatures that had been obtained because of a variety of reasons and as a result the amendment was not on the ballot for Nebraskans to decide in the fall of 2006. The petition organizers may, however, attempt to do so in 2008. Thus, while this is not a new mandated policy for patients, family members, nurses, health care providers, institutions, and other policy and health care actors in the health care system, it is an exemplar case of the intersection of legal and ethical aspects within the context of nursing practice.

Potential Implications for Practice

Had this amendment to the Nebraska state constitution been placed on the November 2006 ballot and voted on by Nebraskans, successfully passed, and became law, Nebraskan nurses would have had to follow the law or face penalties. Their nursing practice with patients in terminal conditions and their respective family members would have been mandated by this state constitutional amendment; the state constitution is the highest law of the state. A nurse who practices in a hospice setting, whether in a hospital, nursing home, or in the home, would be mandated to continue administration of hydration and nutrition by artificial means even if not based in best practice. In this situation the nurse would be compelled to deliver interventions because of the new

Nebraska state law (Nebraskans for Humane Care Committee, 2006). Thus, one can see the tension in decision-making between making decisions based on best practices as in evidence-based practice or decision-making based on the law.

The idea of ethical concerns further complicates the nurse's decision-making process in this Nebraska case study. Nurses must balance their decisions based on what evidence-based practice dictates, what the law mandates, and what the ethical dilemma calls for. For example, perhaps the patient did not want the administration of hydration or nutrition in their particular circumstance but had no expressed advance directive. Without the latter legal document, the patient, family, nurse, other health care providers, nor others in the respective institution could advocate for what the patient may have wanted. Nurses have a responsibility to follow the American Nurses Association (ANA) Code of Ethics. The ANA Code of Ethics can be found at the ANA's Center for Ethics and Human Rights Web site at www.nursingworld.org/ethics. In such a situation, nurses may well fail in their role and responsibility to be advocates for the patient and to advocate for what the patient may have wanted because they fear the penalty of law. Thus, nurses could be violating their own professional ethical code.

What Nurses Need to Know and Do

The Nebraska case study signifies what nurses need to know and what nurses need to do in order to be in control of their profession and to be advocates for their patients. Nurses need to be able to read and understand legal language in order to analyze how that language will affect their practice and conversely their patients. In this case, nurses must know the language of the Nebraska Humane Care Amendment, Section 30, which says (Nebraskans for Humane Care Committee, 2006):

> The fundamental human right to food and water should not be denied to any person, regardless of race, religion, ethnicity, nativity, disability, age, state of health, gender, or other characteristics: No entity with a legal duty of care for a person within its custody (including a hospital, orphanage, foster home, nursing home, sanitarium, skilled nursing facility, prison, jail, detainment center, corporation, business, institution or individual) may refuse, deny, or fail to provide food and water sustenance and nourishment, however delivered, to any such person if death or grave physical harm could reasonably result from such withholding and the person at risk can metabolize. Any such person so threatened with dehydration or starvation, any relative of such person, such person's

legal guardian or surrogate, any public official with appropriate jurisdiction, or any protection and advocacy or ombudsman agency shall have legal standing to bring action for injunctive relief, damages and reasonable attorney's fees to uphold this standard of humane care. This section does not prohibit honoring the will of any person who, by means of a valid advance directive record, has fully expressly, and personally either authorized the withholding of food or water from himself or herself under specific conditions, or delegated that decision, under specific conditions, to one or more relatives or to another person unrelated to the entity with a legal duty of care.

It is important for nurses not only to be attentive to legal language and to understand that language but to critically think about how it affects their decisions. For example, a critique of the language in the proposed amendment reduces the patient to a biological determinant or to a biochemical definition of a human being, especially with the word "metabolize" (Welie, 2006). Aside from the language being reductionistic of a human being, the choice of the word metabolize is incorrect because there is some metabolism after death. It is incongruent with the ethical practice of nurses to practice such reductionistic nursing care. Analysis of other language reflects that minors (and their families) would not have any decision-making rights. When nurses analyze potential laws that interfere with their ability to deliver quality ethical care to patients, they must intervene. Many nurses in Nebraska did exactly that by being part of the coalition group that formed in opposition to this proposed law.

Although most nurses think of laws when the word legal is evoked, the Nebraska case study educates nurses to another important dimension, which is a petition drive to add an amendment to a state constitution, the highest law of one's state. Further, no state law may be in contradiction to constitutional law. This petition drive was promoted by individuals and groups outside of Nebraska. A group, America at Its Best, with a postal address in Kalispell, Montana, was responsible for all of the $835,000 funding for the petition drive for the Nebraska Humane Care Amendment (Stoddard, 2006, August 10). The same group provided almost all of the $861,998 for a second petition drive titled, Stop Over Spending Nebraska, whose purpose was to limit state spending. Of the latter amount, $1,998 was donated by others than the America at Its Best group (Stoddard, 2006, August 10). This group listed the following national organizations as its supporters: Americans for Limited Government, Club for Growth, Funds for Democracy, and the National Taxpayers Union. In Nebraska, 113,721 valid signatures or about 10 percent of registered voters are needed on a petition ballot for it to be voted on at an election (Stoddard, 2006, September 19; Stoddard, 2006,

August 10). The Nebraskans for Humane Care Committee turned in 137,200 signatures.

As noted earlier, nurses need to be able to analyze the use of language by others. Group titles and petition titles can be misleading and/or mean the exact opposite of what a citizen might think the language means. Many Nebraskans signed the petition thinking that the proposed amendment was a "good" thing because the title sounded positive: Who could be against humane care? Eventually, the Nebraska secretary of state found the group did not have enough valid signatures to put the petition on the ballot; about 20 percent of signatures had been declared invalid by county election officials (Stoddard, 2006, September 19). Although this was because of a variety of reasons, one variable will be noted here; individuals who signed were given incorrect and/or fraudulent information when they were asked to sign the petition by the petition seekers. This has ramifications for nurses in their professional and civic lives. When nurses are aware of such misleading or fraudulent behavior on the part of amendment signature seekers, they must be activists. Such policy activity could take several forms: educating their colleagues, family, friends, neighbors; writing letters to the editor of their newspaper; joining coalition groups engaged in the policy issue; and so forth.

Legal Aspects

Nurse Practice Act

One of the most important legal laws affecting nurses is the Nurse Practice Act of their state because that is the law and the legal authority to practice their profession. The Nebraska case study emphasizes the importance of nurses being attentive to legal and ethical dimensions of their practice. This author believes every nurse has been educated and socialized to respect one's nursing license. Nurses know about the necessity of passage of the National Council Licensing Exam for Registered Nurses (NCLEX-RN), of obtaining and maintaining one's nursing license, of knowing the nurse practice act in the state in which one is practicing nursing, knowing and working within one's nursing scope of practice, and of keeping informed about changes in nurse licensure issues. Further, because of living in a litigious society, nurses know the frequency of lawsuits and want to avoid possible loss of their license, termination of their employment, and involvement in a lawsuit as the defendant.

Thus, a core legal aspect for every nurse to know is the importance of their state's nursing practice act. Because the "nursing practice is regulated by each state through a board of nursing established by the state's government" (Wright & DeWitty, 2005, p. 3), nurses must understand what these laws are and how they dictate their practice. A nurse's professional life and economic livelihood is intimately related to the nurse practice act one needs to follow. Violating parts of that act can result in employment and licensure penalties. In every state such a board of nursing has the responsibility and authority to: (1) issue nursing licenses, (2) regulate the practice of nursing, (3) enforce and interpret the specific state's nurse practice act, (4) promulgate administrative law (rules and regulations) which further clarifies the actual law, and (5) discipline nurses as necessary for the goal of ensuring the public's safety in the area of nursing care (Wright & DeWitty, 2005). In addition, a state board of nursing may give advisory opinions to nurses and other interested individuals with questions and concerns about the scope of nursing practice (Wright & DeWitty, 2005).

> Advisory opinions do not have the force or effect of law but generally are issued by a state board in response to evolving issues affecting nursing practice, such as mandatory overtime, or questions related to the scope of practice, such as the peripheral insertion of central venous catheter lines. (p. 4)

For example, in Nebraska there are 36 advisory opinions listed on the Nebraska State Board of Nursing Web site (Nebraska Health and Human Services, n.d.). Examples of advisory opinions on this page that relate to this proposed amendment include such topics as "Abandonment Accountability for Professional Conduct of Nurses." All of these opinions have relevance for the nurses dealing with the proposed Nebraskans for Humane Health Care amendment.

National Council of State Boards of Nursing

Web-based technology and use of the Multistate Nurse Licensure Compact for nurse licensure in many states has increased the helpfulness of the National Council of State Boards of Nursing (NCSBN) for nurses and nurse managers. The NCSBN provides a variety of services to the boards of nursing of all 50 states, the District of Columbia, and the five U.S. territories. These services include (Wright & DeWitty, 2005):

1. Leadership on common concerns
2. Development of the national nursing licensure examination, the NCLEX exam
3. Research and policy analysis
4. Promulgation of national uniformity in the regulation of nursing practice

The technology system established by the NCSBN enables all state boards of nursing to have access to a system of data on nurses' licenses and discipline information. Employees of any state board of nursing can enter or edit data, obtain data on past licensure or license discipline of nurses, and the like. Nursing employers can access this data for a fee. The general lay public cannot access this data. Besides verifying nurses' applicant license information, a board of nursing employee may also use the data system to review disciplinary information of a nurse and to electronically communicate between and among staff at other boards of nursing. This system is especially important given the increased mobility of many individuals and nurses in U.S. society, because of the Multistate Nurse Licensure Compact and the increased use of short-term travel nurses to meet the nursing shortage. Nurses will find the Web site to be a helpful resource. If short-term travel nurses are coming and working in Nebraska, they can use the Web pages of both the National Council of State Boards of Nursing and of Nebraska's state board of nursing to better inform themselves of the kinds of law, policies, and advisory opinions which they must know to practice within their scope of practice in Nebraska.

The NCSBN took a leadership role in the 1990s when they studied and promoted a Multistate Nurse Licensure Compact model for nursing licensure. This model has now been passed by state law in 20 states. See the National Council of State Boards of Nursing Web site for a listing and map of the states that have this model (www.ncsbn.org). This model, based on the driver's license model, allows a nurse to obtain a nursing license in one's state of residency (home state) and to practice in other states (remote states) that also belong to the Multistate Nurse Licensure Compact. The nurse is subject to the nurse practice act of the state in which the nurse is practicing. When practicing in multiple states that belong to the compact, the nurse has one nursing license: that of one's home state (i.e., where one resides). States have to pass laws to join the compact; this is yet another example of how laws and policy affects the practice of nursing.

It is the state board of nursing that addresses any complaints about a nurse; such complaints may trigger the discipline process of that particular state board. Complaints about a nurse could come from a range of individuals: patients, family members, nursing or other work colleagues, employers, or individuals outside the work setting. "The most common complaints filed arise from known or suspected chemical impairment and abuse; drug diversion; criminal convictions; professional boundary violations; and practice deficiencies such as medication errors, documentation discrepancies or the failure to assess or intervene appropriately" (Wright & DeWitty, 2005, p. 6). Although particular practices may vary from one state board of nursing to another, there are the three common steps for a nurse to anticipate after a discipline investigation has been triggered: the board of nursing will conduct an initial investigation, the nurse is informed, then there will be further investigation which results in a range of possible outcomes from dismissal of the complaint to formal charges against the nurse. If a nurse is disciplined, the discipline action could be receiving one of the following:

1. An advisory letter
2. A public reprimand
3. Probation with monitoring by the board of nursing
4. Suspension from nursing practice for a designated time period which may include stipulations for reinstatement
5. Revocation of one's nursing license, either permanently or non-permanently

Because the discipline investigation context is adversarial and because one purpose of a state board of nursing is to protect the public's safety relative to nursing care, nurses are advised to seek legal counsel with an experienced attorney in such an investigative situation.

A state constitution trumps other state laws including a nurse practice act. If the Nebraska case study amendment had been voted on and passed by Nebraskans, nurses (and others) would have to follow that law and/or policy of how one treats all patients in the state. If the nurse chose not to (because of advocacy for the patient determined on evidence-based nursing practice or based on ethical analysis), he or she would be subject to penalty of law—and in conflict with some goals of the nurse practice act administered by the Nebraska State Board of Nursing (to deliver competent, safe care to patients). Further, the nurse would be in conflict with their professional code of ethics and could be in conflict with ethical principles.

Consider now the legal area and its impact on nursing practice using this same Nebraskan case study to understand how law, ethics, and clinical practice are intimately related. It is beyond the purview of this chapter to include all aspects of the law and nursing. Nursing practice is affected by a multitude of federal, state, and city laws, by lawsuits against nurses, by rules and regulations, and by the precedent of court cases. In the following section, we will use the Nebraskan case study to examine how legal issues affect the ethical decision-making process.

Ethical Decision-Making

The significance of the Nebraska case study is found in the stories that nurses tell each other. Nurses experience moral anguish when they engage in ethical dilemmas that concern patient care. While there are many challenges facing nurses in the work environment (nursing shortage, mandatory overtime, and several others), it is the ethical and moral dilemmas that cause the most pain for nurses. The Nebraska case study is only one instance of the kind of frustration, tension, and dilemmas that nurses have. Nurses experience moral anguish with the nursing shortage and knowing that best patient care is not being given. They experience moral anguish when mandated to work overtime—attempting to balance not abandoning their patients with their concern about not giving quality care and their fear of risking a lawsuit because of fatigue and increased risk of medical errors.

In making ethical decisions, three resources that are valuable for nurses are: (1) the ANA Code of Ethics, (2) an understanding of ethical principles, and (3) the ethics of caring. The ANA Code of Ethics was revised in 2001. Although discussion of the code in this part of the chapter concerns ethical dimensions, it also could have been emphasized in the previous legal section of the chapter. For example, if a nurse is involved in a lawsuit, one of the factors that will be analyzed is: Did the nurse follow the ANA Code of Ethics? This is considered a standard of practice. If the nurse did not follow the code of ethics, the nurse's practice is considered substandard.

Historically, a way of understanding ethics in the health system is to study ethics as ethical principles in other words, nonmaleficence, beneficence, fidelity, autonomy versus paternalism, veracity, and justice (Purtilo, 2005). This is the language commonly and routinely read in nursing and health literature, heard when participating in institutional ethics committees, and, the language heard when other nurses and health care providers work through ethical dilemmas. In addition to these, a discussion follows on the ethics of caring which has emerged as another way of solving ethical dilemmas. This latter model comes from the work of Gilligan (1982), other feminists, and nurses.

The principle of *nonmaleficence* is not harming another (Purtilo, 2005). Nurses constantly aim to practice this ethical principle and hold it foremost in their practice. They do not want to harm patients; because nurses are humans, they are healers, they are ethical, and, given one aspect of this chapter, they do not want a lawsuit. Let us reexamine the Nebraskan case study; if there were such a law in Nebraska, nurses would have to choose between following the law and what they know about risks and complications of sustained artificial hydration for dying patients. For example, there is clinical evidence that provision of hydration and nutrition in end-of-life illnesses may cause suffering and may increase aspiration pneumonia and bloating (Post & Whitehouse, 1995). Thus, a law could force nurses to harm a patient. There are a multitude of other examples, where on a daily basis, nurses make decisions, practice preventive interventions, revalidate orders, and use critical thinking and nursing judgment to prevent harm to patients. It can be said that the nurse is the patient's last defense. Nurses' attention to not causing harm to patients has greatly increased the last several years because of the wide professional and lay media coverage of the problem of medical errors in the health care system (Milstead & Furlong, 2006). In a similar way, one chapter of this book includes content on evidence-based nursing because of the concern in the health care system that health providers are not being lifelong learners and applying the latest in best practice health care (Melnyk & Fineout-Overholt, 2005).

The next principle is *beneficence*, which is bringing about good for the patient (Purtilo, 2005). Again, go back to the Nebraskan case study. The proponents and the opponents of the proposed amendment differ on this principle of beneficence. The proponents see this amendment as being positive for the patient. The opponents see other dimensions to the issue, such as it may bring clinical harm to some patients or it violates other ethical principles (patient autonomy, fidelity, justice, etc.). When reflecting on one's nursing practice, the usual situation is that every day that a nurse works, the nurse is making many decisions that are beneficent for the patient. To integrate with legal content discussed earlier in this chapter, the nurse practices beneficent nursing care that meets standards of care and the code of ethics. However, it is easy for the reader to think of many situations for which there can be honest differences of opinion, values, and evaluation of situations in which one person can evaluate that an intervention is harmful and another party sees the intervention as beneficent. This is the ethical dilemma and is the dilemma for this case study. There is a difference of opinion on the beneficence of mandated hydration and nutrition for patients in terminal conditions. Three authors wrote articles during the summer of 2006 analyzing the Catholic moral tradition about end-of-life issues which apply to this case study. One writer, Shannon (2006) "sees the preservation of life at all costs as at least highly troubling, if not as a radical move against the Catholic medical ethics tradition" (p. 29). Drane (2006) analyzes the history of Catholic moral tradition and argues against the provision of artificial nutrition and hydration for all patients. Father Kevin O'Rourke (2006), noted Catholic theologian and ethicist, argues for balancing costs with benefits when making decisions about artificial nutrition and hydration. He stresses the importance of decision-making by the patient, family members, and health providers. His arguments for who should be the decision-makers would be in opposition with the proposed amendment where the state government would be making the decision.

The third principle is *autonomy versus paternalism* (Purtilo, 2005). This means respecting the decision-making of the patient and/or the family members versus only considering the wishes of the health care providers in deciding treatment plans. There has been a paradigm shift in the United States during the past 50-plus years regarding this principle. Prior to about 1950 paternalism by health providers (physicians) was the way decision-making was done. Physicians decided if patients were told certain diagnoses and pressure was put on patients to always follow designated treatments (Friedlander, 1995). This model no longer exists; the emphasis is now on the autonomy of the patient and, by extension, family members. There are many variables to explain this paradigm shift: (1) a U.S. population increasingly educated about their medical conditions, (2) a changed U.S. society where Americans no longer give deference nor authority to several segments of society including the medical system, (3) a changed health care system for which interdisciplinary collaborativeness is recognized as the key to safe patient care versus dominance by physicians, and (4) the reemergence of the U.S. cultural trait of independence.

A current concrete example of this ethical principle of autonomy being practiced can also be seen legally in the federal HIPAA law. One could analyze that particular federal law has emphasized and mandated one aspect of patient autonomy; that of patient decision-making on who will have access to patient information. This third principle applies to the Nebraskan case study. One could argue that the autonomy of patients is not being honored. However, it is not the traditional physician who is being paternalistic; rather, it is out-of-state organizers who are being paternalistic and deciding what is best medically for a population of Nebraska state residents. Had it passed, it would have been the state government being paternalistic in end-of-life decisions. In retrospect, a partial evaluation of why the amendment did not elicit enough signatures in Nebraska integrates with this principle and with some other aspects of the "culture" of Nebraskans. In the United States generally and in some states with a strong politically conservative ideology, there is an antigovernment philosophy; wanting the least amount of governmental intrusion in one's life. Having a state law mandating certain medical treatment violated this Nebraskan philosophy. Another value held by Nebraskans is, if there is going to be government control, then, it should be as local as possible. It was not perceived well by Nebraskans to have change agents from out-of-state fund and attempt to control state policy. At a state population level, Nebraskans do not like this kind of paternalism—whether it is health policy or other policy. Further, such out-of-state tactics is the antithesis of the populist history of this state. In addition to these issues, data from a 2007 survey conducted by the Nebraska Hospice and Palliative Care Organization describes some of the wishes of Nebraskans relative to health care: 33 percent of Nebraskans have an advance directive, and 96 percent "said it's important to be off machines that extend life, and 74 percent wouldn't want medical interventions to keep them alive as long as possible if they were dying" ("Survey Probes," 2007, p. E1). Another data aspect related to this Nebraskan case study is that 75 percent reported they felt total physical dependency on others would be worse than death.

Besides the ethical consideration of autonomy versus paternalism, there is a legal counterpoint to the ethical dimension. The series of lawsuits originating from the classic 1914 lawsuit, Schloendorff v. New York Hospital gave legal power and authority to the individual for what happens to his or her body (*autonomy*) (Menikoff, 2001). Some of these lawsuits also related to the necessity of having informed consent between a health provider and a patient. This third principle of autonomy versus paternalism is deeply rooted both in ethics and the law in this country. The proposed amendment would contradict the history of both ethics and law in this regard.

Nurses in the early twenty-first century recognize the autonomy of patients and family members. If the proposed amendment of the Nebraskan case study had been enacted into law, how would a Nebraska nurse work within this ethical dilemma? Suppose the nurse practices in a hospice setting, the patient has no "fully expressed" advance directive, but the family knows (from many conversations with the dying patient) that he did not want prolonged artificial hydration. What does the nurse do? Follow the law and implement the mandated policy? What about the nurse's responsibility to follow the ethical principle of respecting the patient's autonomy? What about the nurse's responsibility to follow the ANA's Code of Ethics and advocate for patients?

Another ethical principle is that of *justice* (Purtilo, 2005). Justice relates to the nurse's position (professionally and personally) whereby the nurse has the ability to distribute benefits and burdens to individuals and to society. A beginning way to think about the justice imperative is to reflect and evaluate one day in a clinical setting. How did I spend my time? If I was assigned several patients, how did I spend my time? Did I spend it justly? What would be the several patients' perspective, if questioned, of how I divided my time among them? Given the content in all chapters of this book, how would I justify my time with each of them? The reader can think of many more justice issues in nursing. For example, is it just (to patients and to oneself) to continue working on a unit where there is persistent understaffing? Is it just (to patients and to oneself) to continue working in an environment where there is consistent mandatory overtime? There are broader issues in the health care system, such as how should total health care resources be allocated?

There could be many ways to apply this Nebraskan case study to the ethical principle of justice, but just two will be given here. Individuals' behaviors are influenced by many laws and regulations: federal, state, county, and city. The United States—its Constitution and its laws—was forged on a balance between federal and state laws. There is a strong history by Americans of wanting any law or regulation to be at the most local level versus a federal law; the concept of *subsidiarity*. Is it just for individuals outside of one state to make policy for people residing in another state? Is it just to use language—"Nebraskans for a Humane Care Amendment"—

when some individuals would analyze the language as not being totally truthful? Another area of justice relates to cost. Health care costs have always been significant drivers of reform in the system and have affected whether many individuals seek or receive health care. Is it just, from a cost perspective, to mandate sustained hydration and nutrition for all?

In addition to analyzing ethical dilemmas from these four principles, another model to use is that of the ethics of caring. This model of analysis builds on the work of Gilligan and Kohlberg. Over 25 ago, Kohlberg's model of moral development of individuals became the dominant theory. However, Gilligan, one of his graduate students, continued his research—but with girls. She noted differences in how girls, boys, women, and men conceptualized ethical dilemmas (Beauchamp & Childress, 2001; Brannigan & Boss, 2001; Purtilo, 2005). This model of ethical analysis emphasizes relationships, caring for others, listening to others' stories, and balancing justice issues with compassion. While there is not a strict gender division, women tend to embrace a conception of considering the total context of a situation, maintaining and nurturing relationships, and being caring when considering an ethical dilemma. Men tend to evaluate ethical dilemmas more in justice terminology and with more impartial dispassionate conflict resolution.

Because of the dominance of women in the nursing profession, the ethic of care is further emphasized, not only because of the numerical strength of women nurses, but because a core essence of nursing is caring. Health providers and the lay public usually associate caring with nurses and curing with physicians. In the past 25 years, many nurses have written and applied Gilligan's work to nursing. An important aspect of the ethic of caring is narrative ethics requiring "that all voices be considered before the situation is assessed for its moral significance" (Purtilo, 2005, p. 56). In the Nebraskan case study, have all voices been heard?

Nebraska Nurses Respond to the Nebraska Amendment

Nebraska nurses responded and continue to respond to the proposed petition drive that did not get on the ballot in November 2006, using the media to get their points across. For one, Amy Haddad (2006), director of the Center for Health Policy and Ethics (CHPE) at Creighton University, wrote an editorial for the *Omaha World Herald* discussing the issue and raising concerns. For many individuals, this was the first time that concerns with the petition drive were in the public media. Because of the controversy surrounding the issue, Haddad first shared her writing with all levels of university administrators and legal counsel. Second, the Center for Health Policy and Ethics hosted a brown-bag lunch meeting on the issues the amendment raised. Invited speakers included a theology professor, an attorney, and an ethicist from the CHPE who is educated as a physician and attorney as well as an ethicist. Third, the CHPE developed a summary position statement and distributed that statement to attendees. The statement emphasized five areas of concern:

1. Decision-making would be taken from family members and given to the state unless there was a living will with specific language or an appropriate power of attorney.
2. A competent patient could not refuse treatment nor grant or withhold informed consent.
3. The amendment required a procedure that may not help a patient; rather it might cause discomfort and/or hasten death.
4. The amendment proponents presented no evidence of a current concern or problem with patients in Nebraska.

Proponents were presuming that only the use of law and potential legal punishment will assure best care at the end of life. Fourth, a large group of concerned health providers, other individuals, and health agencies formed a coalition to address the concerns they saw with this proposed amendment. This group held many meetings, planned strategies, and educated the public. They recognized that the amendment, while not on the ballot in the fall of 2006 because of technical reasons would most likely be an issue again in the fall of 2008. One example of the kind of education and analysis they did was a lengthy side-by-side column analysis of current law and practice in Nebraska with provisions of the proposed amendment (Anderson, 2006). Analysis by attorney Anderson and others noted the poor legal construction of the proposed amendment because many phrases were vague, language was not defined, and, many phrases were open to interpretation. Another kind of education and analysis was presented by the many nurses who participated in this coalition and who shared their clinical, theoretical, and research knowledge. Many of these nurses were hospice nurses and their knowledge of both dying patients and the literature greatly contributed to others' understanding. In an earlier section of this chapter, it was noted that the petition group, America at Its Best, spent $835,000 on education and lobbying of voters to get on the ballot. Education of health professionals, patients, families, and voters was done on a shoestring budget by the nurses and others discussed in these four responses. This will be a challenge in the summer and fall of 2008 when another petition drive is expected.

The Update of the Nebraska Case Study

As this book goes to press, the Nebraska case study continues. During the spring of 2007, several Nebraska state senators introduced three state laws to address concerns raised by this constitutional amendment and discussed in this chapter. First, Sen. Ray Aguilar introduced Legislative Bill 311 which was unanimously voted out of the Government, Military and Veterans Affairs Committee ("Bills Would," 2007). This bill would change provisions relating to petition signature verification and have such provisions conform to the court case of *Stenberg v. Moore*. The second bill, introduced by Sen. Bill Avery, would change signature thresholds for both constitutional amendments and statutory initiatives ("Bills Would," 2007). His proposed bill, which moved forward from the same unicameral legislative committee by a vote of 6–1, would increase the required number of signatures on constitutional amendments from 10 percent of the state's registered voters to 15 percent. His intent is to make it more difficult to change the state constitution. His and other senators' concerns are the issues discussed in this case study and other petition drives in Nebraska since 1990. Sen. Avery said "I also have deep respect for our state constitution. It deserves to be protected from the desires and whims of out-of-state organizations. It's not written in pencil so that whoever has the biggest eraser can come in and erase it all willy-nilly" ("Bills Would," 2007, p. 7). The third bill, introduced by Sen. DiAnna Schimek, passed the first of three necessary rounds of voting in the full unicameral session by a 31–11 vote on February 1, 2007 (Reed, 2007). This bill would prohibit petition circulators being paid per signature when they are employed for such work. Again, the origin of this bill relates to the concerns and frustrations state senators and others had with the issues discussed in the Nebraska case study. Sen. John Harms' argument during unicameral discussion is reflective of many senators: "That's what got people fired off, it was people coming here from out of state, with no idea about the issues in Nebraska. . . . It was millionaires putting money into telling Nebraskans what to do. That's wrong" (Reed, 2007, B2). In summary, the introduction of these three state laws (with one relying on the judicial outcomes of a court case) demonstrate other important ways that legal decisions affect nursing in addition to constitutional amendments (initiation of state laws and court cases). Nurses in Nebraska are active in lobbying measures on these bills.

Conclusion

Nurses must be cognizant of the many influences that affect decision-making and nurses' decision-making on a daily basis. This book gives the nurse insight into others' decision-making including patients, family members, health care providers, institutional administrators, and policy advocates. While this chapter has focused on some legal and ethical content, the Nebraska case study demonstrated why and how easily one's clinical nursing practice can be significantly altered because of legal activities that may put nurses into legal, ethical, and professional difficulties.

Rentmeester (2006) stated:

> In negotiating uncertainties and responding to interesting, important, and complex questions and dilemmas in healthcare, it appears that healthcare professionals cannot rely solely on legal experts. Rather, they must carefully discern and collegially discuss moral reasons to respond with care to patients and to one another in difficult cases. (p. 32)

The Nebraska case study exemplifies one complex dilemma in patient care: Law; ethics; nurses. They interface with each other in dramatic ways. Nurses need to be prepared for these challenges.

References

Anderson, R., personal communication, September 20, 2006.

Bills would change petition requirements. (2007). *Unicameral Update, XXX*(4), 1, 7.

Beauchamp, T. L., & Childress, J. F. (2001). *Principles of biomedical ethics*. New York: Oxford University Press.

Brannigan, M. C., & Boss, J. A. (2001). *Healthcare ethics in a diverse society*. Mountain View, CA: Mayfield Publishing Company.

Drane, J. F. (2006). Stopping nutrition and hydration technologies: A conflict between traditional Catholic ethics and church authority. *Christian Bioethics, 12*, 11–28.

Friedlander, W. J. (1995). The evolution of informed consent in American medicine. *Perspectives in Biology and Medicine, 38*(3), 498–510.

Gilligan, C. (1982). *In a different voice: Psychological theory and women's development*. Cambridge, MA: Harvard Universtiy Press.

Haddad, A. (2006, July 4). Midlands voices: Health care change would be inhumane. *Omaha World Herald*, Editorial/Opinion page. Retrieved August 10, 2007, from http://chpe.creighton.edu/chpe/focus_fall_2006/owh_opinion.htm

Melnyk, B. M., & Fineout-Overholt, E. (2005). *Evidence-based practice in nursing & healthcare*. Philadelphia: Lippincott Williams & Wilkins.

Menikoff, J. (2001). *Law and bioethics*. Washington, DC: Georgetown Press.

Milstead, J. A., & Furlong, E. (2006). *Handbook of nursing leadership: Creative skills for a culture of safety*. Sudbury, MA: Jones & Bartlett.

Nebraska Health and Human Services. *Advisory opinions*. (n.d.) Retrieved February 23, 2007, from www.hhs.state.ne.us/crl/nursing/Rn-Lpn/advisory.htm

Nebraskans for Humane Care Committee. (2006). *Nebraskans for Humane Care*. Retrieved February 23, 2007, from www.nehumanecare.com

O'Rourke, K. (2006). Reflections on the papal allocution concerning care for persistent vegetative state patients. *Christian Bioethics, 12*, 83–97.

Post, S., & Whitehouse, P. (1995). Fairhill guidelines on ethics of the care of people with Alzheimer's disease: A clinical summary. *Journal of the American Geriatrics Society, 43*, 1423–1429.

Purtilo, R. (2005). *Ethical dimensions in the health professions* (4th ed.).
    Philadelphia: Elsevier Saunders.

Reed, L. (2007, February 2). Petition restrictions advance. *Omaha World Herald*,
    p. B1–2.

Rentmeester, C. A. (2006). What's legal? What's moral? What's the difference?
    A guide for teaching residents. *American Journal of Bioethics, 6*(4), 31–32.

Shannon, T. A. (2006). Nutrition and hydration: An analysis of the recent
    papal statement in the light of the Roman Catholic bioethical tradition.
    Christian Bioethics, 12, 29–41.

Stoddard, M. (2006, August 10). Outsiders fueled two petition drives. *Omaha
    World Herald*, p. B1–2.

Stoddard, M. (2006, September 19). Humane care vote could be in '08.
    Omaha World Herald, p. A1.

Survey probes attitudes on death, dying. (2007, February 5). *Omaha World
    Herald*, p. E1.

Wright, L. D., & DeWitty, V. P. (2005). *Legal basics for professional nursing practice.*
    Silver Springs, MD: Center for American Nurses.

Welie, J., personal communication, October 23, 2006.

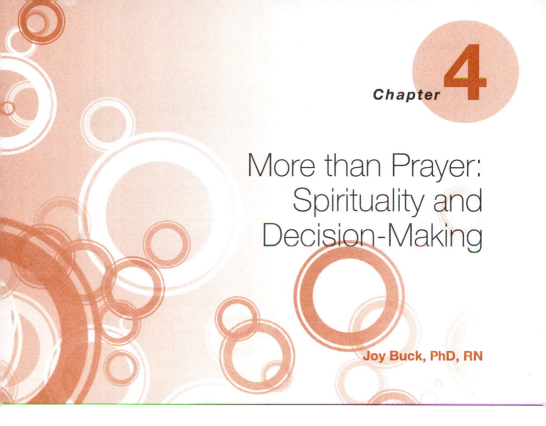

Chapter 4

More than Prayer: Spirituality and Decision-Making

Joy Buck, PhD, RN

When Hannah was diagnosed with a progressive and fatal neurological disorder, she was 3 years old. Within 2 months of her diagnosis, she was admitted to a local hospice program. Concurrent with Hannah's rapid decline, her mother Ruth learned that she was pregnant. During her first prenatal visit, her OB/GYN recommended an amniocentesis and an abortion if the fetus carried the genetic trait for the disease. Until this point, neither Ruth nor her husband believed that they would ever consider an abortion—yet, as they watched Hannah struggle, it was difficult for them to fathom going through this process again and subjecting another child to the suffering that Hannah experienced. They had to choose whether to go through with the amniocentesis and if they did, what action they would take if the results for the genetic trait were positive.

When the hospice intake nurse visited to assess Hannah's condition and the parents' readiness for hospice, she explained that, although the hospice typically took care of terminally ill adults, two of their hospice nurses, Tina and Susan, had pediatric experience. Tina worked full-time and volunteered to be the primary nurse with Susan, a part-time employee, serving as the backup. After the intake visit and prior to Tina's first visit, the hospice team discussed Hannah's case and how best to support the parents in their dilemma. It was during this discussion that the social worker suggested that Tina remove the antiabortion button she wore on her purse prior to entering Hannah's home. Tina countered that she could not do that because she believed that she had a religious obligation to preserve life at all costs. By contrast, the social worker suggested that Hannah's parents were already having a difficult time and that wearing the button into the home would be insensitive at best. Although the hospice's executive director shared Tina's beliefs, she also believed that Tina had a professional obligation to be objective and not impose her religious views on Hannah's parents. She decided that because Tina could not in good conscience remove the button from her purse that Susan should be the primary nurse and another nurse would serve as backup.

Over the next 2 weeks, Susan and the hospice social worker made frequent visits to assess Hannah's condition and parental coping. During these visits, they helped the parents reflect on their situation, clarified their conceptions and misconceptions, and explored the pros and cons of their options. In doing so, they assisted the parents to understand that they were the ones who would live with the consequences of their decision and as such, they should make their decision based on their beliefs. They could choose whether to have the amniocentesis as well as their course of action if the test were positive. In the end, although they couldn't imagine the thought of losing another child to the disease, they also couldn't choose to have an abortion if the test were positive. After a great deal of soul searching, they decided not to have the amniocentesis and found another OB/GYN who could support them with their decision.

This scenario reflects the extent to which diverse religious and spiritual beliefs shape personal and clinical decision-making in distinct ways. In this case, a physician recommended both testing and a specific course of action. She made that recommendation based on her belief that it would be unethical to not test for the genetic marker or to allow the pregnancy to continue if the test came back positive. The parents were not religious but deeply spiritual and her recommendation was in conflict with their values. They were in crisis and experiencing the loss of one child while considering the fate of another. Turning to their faith in a higher power, they achieved a sense of equanimity with their decision and ability to handle whatever came their way. The hospice team, two of whom held similar religious beliefs, interpreted the situation through different cultural, religious, and spiritual lenses. The team openly discussed the best way to proceed from a variety of perspectives. Although Tina continued to hold her strong beliefs, her coworkers respected her right to them while assuring compassionate care for Hannah and her family. By assisting the parents to process their beliefs and to weigh the benefits and risks of their options in an empathic and objective manner, Susan and the social worker helped them to come to terms with the situation in front of them and to develop a sense of balance during an emotionally tumultuous time.

Spirituality and Decision-Making Defined

Historically, faith traditions have played a dominant role in the development of the nursing profession (O'Brien, 1999; Shelley & Miller, 1999). Today, there is consensus that greater attention should be given to the spiritual dimensions of nursing care, but there is no clear direction about what spiritual care is or under what circumstances it is appropriate or desirable. The term *spirituality* means different things to different people. The literature suggests that classifications of spirituality range from the strictly religious to the strictly secular (van Leeuwen, Tiesinga, Post, & Jochemsen, 2006). In the case study, Tina made her decision based on the basis of a religious doctrine that values life at all costs. This is consistent with the traditional definition of spirituality as ". . . something that in ecclesiastical law belongs to the church or to a cleric" (Merriam-Webster's, 2003). Hannah's parents made their decision based on their interpretation of spirituality as a quest for meaning that in their case was not associated with religious beliefs, rituals, or practices.

While no common definition of spirituality exists, nurse authors and theorists have explored the meaning of spirituality in nursing practice (Buck, 2007; Humphreys, 2001; McSherry & Cash, 2004; Tanyi, 2002; Post-White et al., 1996). When combined, definitions of spirituality include the elements of transcendence, mystery, connectedness, meaning and purpose, hope, higher power, and relationships (Tanyi, 2002; van Leeuwen et al., 2006). Some researchers have found Antonovsky's Salutogenic Model of Health (1979) and central construct, sense of coherence (SOC) useful. This model posits that sense of coherence is essential to wellness. *Sense of coherence* is defined as being a dynamic process through which one finds meaning and understanding in life events, and perceives that there are resources available to help confront the situation (Antonovsky, 1979). A sense of coherence is conceptually similar to hope. In a study of hopefulness in cancer patients, the authors identified five central themes that increased sense of coherence and quality of life in participants, including finding meaning and having affirming relationships (Post-White et al., 1996). McSherry and Cash (2004) proposed a taxonomy of spirituality that included the following descriptors: theistic, or a belief in a supreme being or deity; religious, a belief in God and certain religious practices, rituals, and customs; language, including expressions of inner peace and strength; social, political, and cultural ideologies; phenomenological, the process of learning through experiences; existential, a semantic philosophy of life and being; quality of life; and, mystical, the relationship between transcendent, interpersonal and transpersonal.

This chapter uses a broad definition of spirituality as a personal search for meaning that may or may not be related to religion as a basis to explore the relevance of spiritual beliefs in end-of-life decision-making from the perspective of nurses, patients, and families. The term *religious* will be used for specific religious practices and values. Beginning with an examination of the historical relevance of spirituality to nursing care, this chapter uses a series of case studies to investigate how spiritual and religious beliefs shape individual perceptions, interpretations, and interactions among and between health professionals, patients, and their families. The chapter concludes with recommendations and resources to assist nurses to understand their own spirituality and values while appreciating those of their patients, families, and communities.

Rites and Rights of Living and Dying

The issues of medical beneficence, quality of life, and respect for the sanctity of life have been described in medical and philosophical writings since the earliest documented history. The questions central to these issues have remained constant throughout history, but advances in scientific knowledge and technology continually reframe our understanding of both the questions and answers. Throughout history, debates have proliferated around the question of locus of control over one's ultimate destiny. These discussions have centered on such issues as the degree of human suffering, public and military utility, economics, presence of terminal illness, lunacy, and/or fear of dishonor (Humphrey & Wickett, 1986). The understanding of when an individual has the right—whether legal or moral—to assert control changes in the context of time and place.

Until the middle of the twentieth century, care for the dying was firmly within the domain of home, family, and religion (Buck, 2007; Buhler-Wilkerson, 2001; Smith & Nickel, 1999). Family members, primarily women, would care for the dying person and prepare the body for burial when they died. For those with financial means, private nurses were hired to care for the dying person. The terminally ill without family or financial means to pay for care in voluntary hospitals were sent to almshouses or asylums until they died—or in some circumstances they were cared for in specialized homes for the dying. Many of these homes, though not all, were founded by groups of the Christian and Jewish faiths. These groups varied in their approaches to management of the death bed and rituals prior to and after death—yet, they were bound to a commitment to religious ideals and beliefs that called them to serve the most vulnerable in their midst (Clark, 1997; Humphreys, 2001; Siebold, 1992; Walsh, 1929).

By the late 1940s, a series of social, political, and economic forces resulted in an expansion of the role of the federal government in health care and served to further institutionalize and professionalize care for the dying. Federal funding, especially after World War II bolstered the medical system through funding for hospitals, medical and nursing education, and the advancement of medical science and technology. The resultant increase in the number of hospital beds and capacity for "life saving" was due, in part, to other changes in society such as the mobility of the population, the transference of the extended family to the nuclear family, and women's work outside the home (Buck, 2005). The transition of care for the dying from home to hospital had a profound impact on the process of dying and the important role of family and religion within that process.

As the locus of care and control over death changed, the context of the dying moved from the moral to technical order. Cassel (1974) characterized death in the moral order as a process that allowed for "caring for" and rituals to ease the passage of the mortal body to the immortal soul. In contrast, death in the technical order was a definitive event marked by cessation of certain biological functions. The focus was not on the person or spirit, but rather on the science and technology of the measurement of organ function. Dying in the technical order reduced death to a series of technical events that accompany biological function and indicated the end of life. Death initially was defined as the cessation of heartbeat and respiration. The emergence of organ transplantation and medical technology to measure brain waves resulted in a change of the definition of death from the heart and lungs to the brain to allow for the harvesting of organs from brain-dead individuals. Whereas at one time death was once considered a natural occurrence, its medicalization transformed it into a distinctly unnatural event.

During the 1960s, research funded by the U.S. Public Health Service Division of Nursing documented the stark realities of institutionalized dying: Pain control was virtually nonexistent and terminally ill cancer patients frequently died in a room at the end of the hall, in exquisite pain and alone (Duff & Hollingshead, 1968; Glaser & Strauss, 1965, 1968; Quint, 1967; Sudnow, 1967). Social movements outside the walls of medical institutions began to clamor for the reform of care provided within. The civil and women's rights, death with dignity, and consumer movements laid a foundation for a growing public discourse about the quality of life, patients' rights, and the place of informed consent in the medical system. Stories of how cancer patients suffered while undergoing aggressive curative treatment were widely publicized in the popular press. Despite the promise of curative medicine, many began to wonder if the quest for cure was worth the human toll in suffering (Buck, 2005).

Although there were many people involved with the death and dying movements that emerged during the twentieth century, it was

American psychiatrist Elisabeth Kübler-Ross who played a pivotal role in stimulating serious reforms. She helped revolutionize society's conceptualization of death, dying, and bereavement with the publication of her book *On Death and Dying* in 1969. In this book, she described what dying patients commonly felt: "I am in pain, I feel tired, I'm lonely." She decried the kind of institutionalized care given to the dying when she wrote: "He may cry for rest, peace, and dignity, but he will get infusions, transfusions, a heart machine, or tracheotomy if necessary" (Kübler-Ross, 1969, p. 9). Despite her critics, and there were many, Kübler-Ross' writings reached international lay and professional audiences. In the early 1970s, nurses commonly cited Kübler-Ross as having the greatest influence on their attitudes toward death, and by 1976, her book had sold more than a million copies. Journalists attributed Kübler-Ross as single-handedly turning around an entire generation of opinion makers on the topic (Filene, 1998).

In the mid-1970s, media coverage of the Karen Anne Quinlan case further propelled the "right-to-die movement" into the collective American consciousness and the movement from incipiency into coalescence. The landmark Quinlan case revolved around a family's wish to withdraw life-sustaining medical intervention, specifically a ventilator, from Karen Anne because she was deemed to be in a persistent, vegetative state. The decision in this case was not based on her brain or organ death, or extreme suffering, but rather on the basis of the quality of her life. Was living in a persistent vegetative state a life that should be sustained? Public debate on this issue was centered on questions about an individual's right to self-determination, the rights of surrogates acting on behalf of others, determinations of the quality and futility of life, the conditions under which one might choose to end life, and protections for those who helped them die in the manner they chose; all issues that we continue to debate today (Buck, 2005; Filene, 1998; Webb, 1997).

It was within this context that the hospice movement emerged and nurses were critical to its vitality in the United States. Florence Wald, the acknowledged hospice midwife in the United States, was dean of the Yale School of Nursing when she first heard British physician Cicely Saunders speak about hospice in 1963. The hospice ideal resonated to the core of Wald's being and she made a commitment to transplant Saunders' vision of hospice onto U.S. soil (Buck, 2004; Krisman-Scott, 2001). Unlike Cicely Saunders, who cited her evangelistic Christian faith as being foundational to her commitment to the care of the terminally ill, Wald was motivated by a deep sense of moral obligation to humanity and social justice (Buck, 2005; Clark, 1998; du Boulay, 1984). She found a strong ally in Reverend Edward Dobihal, an evangelistic Methodist minister with a background in pastoral counseling and bereavement. Together, they initiated a multidisciplinary effort to research and reform care for the dying. In 1971, they, along with a growing group of supporters, founded a nonprofit organization, Hospice, Inc. By 1974, the group had funding to open the first modern hospice home care program and hospice was well on its way to becoming a national phenomenon and a reimbursable model of care under the Medicare program (Buck, 2004; 2005).

Although the hospice movement cut across many societal boundaries and challenged assumptions about the appropriate care for the dying, serious inadequacies exist in the contemporary models of care at the end of life. As medical and technological advances provide more treatment options, societal debates over the moral implications of treatment withdrawal have become increasingly contentious and polarized. Evidence of this can be seen in the Terri Schiavo case (Allen, 2005; Annas, 2005; Cerminara, 2005; Cohen, 2006; Fins, 2006; Ganzini, 2006; Johnson, 2006; Marks, 2005; Paris, 2006; Perry, 2006; Roscoe, Osman, & Haley, 2006; Schwarz & Coyle, 2006; Wolfson, 2005). Nurses were in the thick of this controversy and are often involved with the care of individuals and families in crisis. As such, it is important that they reflect on their own spirituality and how their beliefs shape interactions with their colleagues, patients, and families entrusted to their care.

This brief historical overview provides insights into the significance of religious and secular ideals to twentieth-century terminal care reform efforts. The connection between the religious call to care for the dying is most explicitly demonstrated with the evolution of religious homes for the dying in the United States, some of which are still operational (Buck, 2006). As hospice struck a responsive chord in the United States, research revealed that when compared to nurses in standard settings, hospice nurses were characterized as having deep spiritual faith and a well-developed commitment to finding meaning in life through service to others (Amenta, 1984; Pannier, 1980). Many of the early hospice training programs for staff and volunteers focused on the highly philosophical notions of the meaning of life and death, "being with," ministering to and caring for dying patients and their families. These groups faced challenges in determining what spiritual care meant in a religiously plural society—yet, these discussions led to the reintroduction of spirituality as an explicit and essential component of care for the terminally ill (Buck, 2005; 2007).

Spirituality and Decision-Making in Contemporary Times

Although it is clear that deeply held spiritual beliefs shaped career and end-of-life care decisions in the past, in what ways do they shape these issues today? Spiritual faith has been shown to be a protective factor during times of transitions and crisis. It is important to note, however, that religiosity is not necessarily synonymous with having faith or being spiritual. In some circumstances, religiosity has been associated with damaging or deleterious effects as well (Strawbridge, Shema, Cohen, Roberts, & Kaplan, 1998).

There is considerable variation in how individuals perceive and act on their beliefs at the end of life. Many hospice and palliative care professionals have developed expertise in assessing and providing spiritual care at the end of life, or at least referring patients for such care. Still, people die across the lifespan and across care settings and many people choose not to access hospice and palliative care services during the last years of their lives. Nurses are frequently in a position to facilitate treatment decisions; thus, it is important for all nurses to consider the ways in which spirituality influences making decisions about advance directives (AD), treatment withdrawal, and the use of advanced technology to sustain life.

Spiritual Faith and Hope

Americans are for the most part religious. In a religiously plural society such as the United States, the meanings and expressions of religious and spiritual faith are diverse. Recent research reveals that 9 of 10 Americans believe in God or a "higher power" and over two thirds of them use prayer as a source of comfort (Gallup & Lindsay, 1999; Okon, 2005). In one study, the majority of respondents described themselves as being both religious and spiritual; 10 percent characterized themselves as being spiritual but nonreligious (Shahabi, Powell, Musick, Pargament, Thoresen, & Williams, 2002). Several studies suggest that medical professionals are far less religious or spiritual than the general public. One study found that family physicians' religious and spiritual beliefs were comparable to the general population, but only 39 percent of psychiatrists agreed that religious faith was an important part of their lives (Bergan & Jensen, 1990). Additional studies suggest that this disparity might not be as pronounced as once thought. In sum, the extent of health professionals' spiritual and religious beliefs and the influence of these beliefs in clinical decision-making have not been firmly established. Recent trends in procreative rights suggest an increasing number of pharmacists and physicians are refusing to fill and write prescriptions for what is called "Plan B," or in some cases, birth control pills. These decisions are made on the basis of religious beliefs that life begins at conception and that life must be preserved at all costs (Gee, 2006).

Spirituality, Risk, and Resiliency

Spiritual belief has been shown to provide social support, hope, and a mechanism to aid in coping with the fragility of life (Daugherty et al.,

2004; Feher & Maly, 1999; Koenig, 2004; Taylor, 2006). In a study of the influence of spiritual beliefs in patients with advanced cancer, the authors found little association between patients' spiritual or religious problem-solving style and awareness of their prognosis or decision-making process. The study participants elected to enter the clinical trials because, in the words of one patient: "I put faith in doctors and God" (Daugherty et al., 2004, p. 141). This study found that spirituality was not associated with more or less realism about prognosis, but that it might play an important role in the patients' ability to be both optimistic and hopeful. In essence, faith offers a mechanism by which patients could be simultaneously realistic while still maintaining hope in a miracle. Similar to this study, other studies have shown that those entering clinical trials have faith in the anticancer effects of the experimental treatments, despite the low likelihood that they would be effective (Hutchinson, 1998).

Spiritual beliefs play a significant role in deciding whether to have genetic testing. As was the case with Hannah's parents, spiritual individuals tend to be more optimistic, more likely to attribute disease to external forces versus genetic ones, and have greater acceptance with certain diagnoses, such as cancer (Ellison & Levin, 1998; Jenkins & Pargament, 1995). In a study of women at high risk for breast cancer, the authors found that influence of faith in genetic testing decisions, in this case BRCA1/1 testing, was dependent on a woman's perception of risk versus religious beliefs (Schwartz et al., 2000). Other studies conducted on spirituality and health risk behaviors among adolescents and pregnant women show a positive correlation between spiritual well-being and reduced health risk-taking behavior. It is important to understand the distinctions between religion and spiritual well-being. Research in adolescents has shown positive correlations between depression and high risk-taking behavior (Albrecht, Reynolds, Cornelius, Heidinger, & Armfield, 2002; Cotton, Larkin, Hoopes, Cromer, & Rosenthal, 2005; Lerher, Shrier, Gortmaker, & Buka, 2006; Shapiro, Radecki, Charchian, & Josephson, 1999). One study identified that most of the adolescents reported some connection with religious and spiritual concepts. Adolescents with higher levels of spiritual well-being, in this case measured as level of existential well-being, had fewer depressive symptoms and fewer risk-taking behaviors. This study supported the need to move beyond an examination of religious identification or attendance at religious services to broader concepts of spirituality (Cotton et al., 2005). Although this mechanism is not fully understood, several studies on depression in female caregivers demonstrate that religiosity was associated with feelings of "role burden" that resulted in increased symptoms of depression (Leblanc, Driscoll, & Pearlin, 2004) In addition, Pargament and colleagues (1995; 1996) found that the use of religion as a coping mechanism, in some instances, encourages people to impose their religious views on others, interpersonal rigidity and/or to view their suffering as something that is deserved and must be endured (Pargament, Van Haitsma, & Ensing, 1995). Tina's response to being asked to remove the antiabortion pin from her purse is one example of this.

The following story about Carroll offers an example of how dissonance between one's religious beliefs and behavior shape interpretations of the meaning of disease. Carroll was 38 and had three children when he confessed to his wife that he had been having sexual affairs with men. He told her that he still loved her and the children and hoped that they could stay together, but he could not keep his sexual orientation a secret any longer. His wife was devastated and could not comprehend how he could do this to her. Their religion viewed homosexuality as a sin and she asked him to go to reparative therapy to cure him. Carroll also believed that his sexual attraction to men was a sin and he agreed to enter a program. The program was not effective and Carroll was left feeling that he had failed everyone, including God. His wife divorced him and he moved from the southern town where he had been raised to live in Washington, DC.

Ten years later, Carroll became sick and tests revealed that he was in the advanced stages of HIV disease. He was put on five different medications to help contain the virus and prevent opportunistic infections from developing. The nurse practitioner was very clear about his need to follow the drug regimen closely and he promised that he would. He was also referred to a local HIV/AIDS community-based organization (CBO). He grew particularly close to Kathy, one of the CBO's volunteers. She visited Carroll frequently and one afternoon she noticed a pile of unfilled prescriptions on his desk. When she asked why he hadn't filled them, he said that they were too expensive. She reminded him that his private insurance plan covered the cost of the medications and asked him what the real reason was. Carroll then told her that he brought this disease on himself and that it was wrong for him to use his insurance to pay for the consequences of his mistakes. There was nothing that Kathy or anyone else involved with Carroll's care could do or say to disavow him of the belief that his disease was God's retribution for his sins.

Spirituality and Individual and Familial Decision-Making

Since 1972, when the Death with Dignity Act (DDA) became law in the United States, the legal and clinical context of decision-making at the end of life has changed considerably. Both the DDA and more recent Patient Self Determination Act of 1991 were enacted, in part, based on the assumption that power and control over life and death decisions should be vested in the individuals who would be most impacted by these decisions rather than professionals. Individual autonomy over choosing one's own ultimate destiny continues to be an important motivator for those completing advanced directives—yet, many Americans do not have them for a variety of reasons. Deeply embedded cultural and spiritual beliefs shape individual perceptions of what constitutes a good death and who should be in charge of decision-making in regard to treatment in distinctly different ways (True, Phipps, Braitman, Harralson, Harris, & Tester, 2005).

Several studies have demonstrated that racial differences in advance care planning and requests for aggressive medical care in terminally ill patients exist. When compared to Caucasians, African Americans are less likely to have any form of advance directive and more likely to request hospitalization and aggressive life-sustaining measures regardless of prognosis (Caralis, Davis, Wright, & Marcial, 1993; Johnson, Elbert-Avila, & Tulsky, 2005). These differences have been attributed to distrust of the health care system, economic disparities, and cultural beliefs about what constitutes "optimal" care for the dying. While these variables are certainly valid, an individual's spiritual belief is an important variable as well (Caralis et al., 1993; Garrett, Harris, Norburn, Patrick, & Danis, 1993; Johnson et al., 2005; True et al., 2005). The following case study examines the impact of race and spiritual beliefs on the willingness of family members to forego life-sustaining treatments.

Mary was a 66-year-old African American woman with diabetes, hypertension, and early dementia who lived with her husband of 40 years. One afternoon, her husband Leonard came home to find her unconscious on the floor and called for an ambulance to take her to the hospital. An MRI showed a large arteriovenous malformation had caused an intercerebral hemorrhage and she was taken to the operating room for its repair. Although the surgeons were successful in stopping the bleeding, during the postoperative period, she remained unconscious and only responded to painful stimuli by opening her eyes. When the surgeons told the husband of her poor prognosis and suggested palliative care, he refused stating: "It's in God's hands now . . . he'll take her home when he's ready." Over the next few weeks, the clinical staff became increasingly frustrated over his refusal to remove life support. They called for a palliative care consultation to help the staff work with the husband and it proved fruitful. With the assistance of Leonard's and Mary's minister, he was able to bridge hope for a miracle to the reality that she would not survive. She was taken off the ventilator and died peacefully with her husband and minister by her side.

Keeping in mind that applying broad generalizations about any population or group is problematic, this case study supports the growing body of research about racial differences in spiritual beliefs and practices. In a comprehensive review of the literature of spirituality and end-of-life decision-making in African Americans, the authors noted four concurrent themes (Johnson et al., 2005). The first theme related to the significance of spiritual practices, particularly prayer as a coping mechanism in times of illness. The second was related to the practice of giving their troubles to God and faith in prayer as a pathway to healing. The third theme was a belief that one's fate was in the hands of God, not man. The fourth related theme was the belief that God used physicians as an "instrument of healing" (Johnson et al., 2005). These themes are also evident in other populations and when controlling for race and ethnicity, the most salient variable is religious faith. Interestingly, one study showed that religiosity in nurses was negatively correlated with ease in death and dying situations (Wortham, 1989). These findings suggest a paradox in an individual's profession of faith and trusting in God's will while at the same time clinging to artificial means to prolong life and discomfort when caring for dying patients is interesting and worthy of much greater study.

While spiritual and religious beliefs are often associated with the prolongation of life-sustaining treatments, the converse is true as well. In regard to treatment preferences at the end of life, a significant barrier to hospice care among African Americans of faith is their belief that only God has the power to decide whether someone should live or die. As such, advance directives or choosing to enter a hospice program is contrary to their religious beliefs (Jackson, Schim, & Seely, 2000; Johnson et al., 2005; Reesek, Ahren, & Nair, 1999). For example, in one study participants commented that ". . . only God should end someone's suffering. . . . God is able to send cures for all illness, terminal or otherwise" (Johnson et al., 2005, p. 713). Moreover, a rare study examining nurses' attitudes toward assisted suicide revealed a positive correlation between the religiosity of nurses and a positive attitude toward assisting patients in their requests for assistance in ending their lives (Matzo, 1996). Although this study found that nurses were more inclined to discuss their decisions to assist a patient with physicians, they did not discuss them with their colleagues or supervisors. Thus we see that spiritual faith and decision-making is complex and variable and that it is important to assess individual religious views and how these are translated into clinical decision-making.

Conflicting Views: Spiritual Dissonance

Thus far, this chapter has focused primarily on the ways that spiritual beliefs are related to clinical decision-making by patients and their families. These decisions are not made in isolation, however, and often nurses are required to carry out treatments that are in contrast to their own beliefs. The following case study published in the neonatal literature offers a careful examination of the ethical and spiritual conflicts that arise between health professionals and families (Stutts & Schloemann, 2002). In this scenario, a premature African American infant developed mild respiratory distress syndrome and was intubated soon after birth. Over the next several months, the infant experienced a series of complications, including severe respiratory distress, disseminated intravascular coagulation, septicemia, necrosis of the bowel, and renal failure. When the staff discussed the infant's poor prognosis with the parents, they said that the infant's ". . . outcome was in God's hands" and they refused to redirect care from aggressive to palliative intervention.

As the infant's condition continued to deteriorate, the staff grew increasingly uncomfortable with continuing aggressive therapies and asked for legal and ethical consults about their options. The hospital chaplain and members of the ethics committee spoke with the parents and as they did, the parents became more resistant and distrustful. Ultimately, the infant died 152 days after birth and the staff who cared for him went through a series of debriefing sessions. In the end, the spiritual and cultural conflicts that arose between the staff and parents made it difficult for the professionals to provide what they believed to be optimal care for the infant. Although the debriefing sessions were useful, the authors conclude by emphasizing how the situation might have been prevented if the staff had spent more time considering the situation through the social, cultural, and spiritual lens of the parents (Stutts & Schloemann, 2002).

In this scenario, the professionals viewed issues of bioethics and quality of life quite differently than the parents. The resultant dissonance resulted in the parents becoming increasingly defensive and suspicious of the professionals. At the same time, the staff became increasingly anguished about having to prolong what they perceived to be suffering in the infant. In this case, the hospital was proactive in supporting the staff by providing time to debrief and express their frustration in an open and nonjudgmental manner. Although these group meetings did not totally diffuse the situation, they did provide a venue for the staff to receive support and express their concerns. This case study reveals how disparate views about the appropriate care of terminally ill children impact the experiences of dying and loss. The staff did not fully understand the deep and profound sense of loss the parents were experiencing. Although the staff dealt with these issues on a daily basis and desired to end the infant's suffering, the parents were naïve to such situations. Professional discussions of medical futility and explanations of the findings of ethics committees did little to support them and, in fact, served to alienate them. In trying to do what the staff deemed the best for the infant, they failed to provide the type of supportive care the parents needed during this time of crisis. If they had fully considered the parents' perspective and responded accordingly, they might well have been able to help the parents in their grief.

Moral Distress and Decision-Making Among Professionals

It is important for health care professionals to consider another person's point of view. It is equally important that they reflect upon their own beliefs. Many times intra- and interprofessional and interpersonal conflicts arise but the true source of the conflict is never identified. In the case studies presented so far in this chapter, difficulties arise when there is a dissonance between patient and familial values and worldviews and that of health professionals. The literature on the role of faith in medical decision-making among health professionals is limited. The research that does exist suggests that faith is not an important factor in physician and nurse decision-making (Okon, 2005). Still, as we saw in the neonatal case study, nurses often experience "moral distress" when they are required to "act in a manner which violates personal beliefs and values about what is right and wrong" (Fenton, 1988). Moral distress has been found to be a significant source of emotional suffering in nurses and anecdotally associated with job dissatisfaction, decreased quality patient care, and implicated in nurses leaving the workforce (Nathaniel, 2002). Thus, it behooves health professionals to critically examine the sources and implications of moral distress in the clinical arena and to develop preventive measures, as well as interventions to reduce the negative effects of moral distress when it occurs. The following case study examines an all-too-familiar story in intensive care units across the country.

Kate was a nurse working in a medical/surgical intensive care unit in a community hospital. Although Kate enjoyed working with critically ill cardiac patients, over time she grew dismayed by the medical management of other patients in the unit. Several physicians continued aggressive therapies and advanced life support in terminally ill patients. It was morally incomprehensible to her that patients and their families were not told the truth about their conditions or included in treatment decisions. She began to advocate on behalf of these patients and honestly answer questions about the patients' conditions and treatments when asked. Although the families were grateful for her help, several of her coworkers were uncomfortable with her doing this without the physician's permission.

When a 50-year-old patient with lung cancer was admitted to the ICU unit, Kate was at a breaking point. The patient had been diagnosed with inoperable lung cancer 6 months prior to his admission and recently had been referred to a hospice program. Within a few weeks he developed respiratory distress and a fever and opted to go to the emergency room for antibiotics. Although he didn't want to be resuscitated in the event of pulmonary arrest, he did agree to be admitted to the hospital for IV antibiotic therapy. The day after his admission, he stopped breathing and a code was called despite his wife's protestations. A pulmonologist who did not know the patient but responded to the code convinced her that he could cure the pneumonia. The patient was intubated, placed on a respirator, and sent to the ICU where Kate took care of him for the next 3 weeks. As it turned out, the man had developed a necrotizing pneumonia that was nonresponsive to antibiotic therapy. As his condition continued to decline, it became increasingly clear to everyone except the pulmonologist that further treatment was medically futile and would cause undue suffering. The man was alert and was willing to continue therapy until his wife was ready to let him go. Kate was becoming enmeshed in the situation and requested a different patient assignment; it was denied. When Kate asked the supervisor to bring the case up at the ethics committee, the supervisor said that the physician had the right to direct the patient's care and refused.

The next morning, Kate decided to take things into her own hands. When she spoke to the man's wife, Kate learned that the wife was wracked with guilt about allowing his resuscitation. Kate explained that despite the mechanical ventilation, he wasn't getting enough oxygen to sustain organ function. His kidneys were failing and he was filling up with fluid. The pulmonologist called the nephrologist who recommended dialysis. When Kate discussed the pros and cons of this with the wife, the wife responded: "I let go of him once. I'm not sure that I can let go of him again"—yet, at the same time neither she nor her husband wanted him to linger and watching him suffer was becoming more than she could bear. At the wife's request, Kate called the hospital chaplain for pastoral counseling. That afternoon while Kate was at lunch, the man had a cardiac arrest and when she returned to the unit, resuscitation efforts were underway. The patient did not respond and when Kate called the pulmonologist for permission to discontinue the code, he refused. Two other ICU nurses continued to work the code; Kate supported the man's wife while she called family. At the end of the shift, Kate gave her supervisor 2-weeks notice and vowed to never work in a hospital again.

Kate's story is not an unusual one. A growing body of literature examining the source and manifestations of moral distress in nurses demonstrates that the continuation of futile care often evokes strong emotional responses from nurses (Ferrell, 2006). Psychologists define moral distress as the state experienced when moral choices and actions are thwarted by constraints (Austin, Rankel, Kagan, Bergum, & Lemermeyer, 2005). Moral dilemmas among nurses arise due to a variety of factors, including institutional demands, interpersonal and intraprofessional conflicts, and interdisciplinary disputes. The intensity of moral distress and work environment has been linked to the frequency of moral distress experienced by nurses. One study suggests a negative correlation of age and moral distress intensity and that being African American was related to higher levels of moral distress intensity (Corley, Minick, Elswick, & Jacobs, 2005). In critical care nurses, the frequency of moral distress situations that are perceived as futile or nonbeneficial to their patients has a significant relationship to the experience of emotional exhaustion, a main component of burnout (Meltzer & Huckabay, 2004).

Moral distress among nurses has far-reaching implications. Moral distress adversely affects job satisfaction, retention, psychological and physical well-being, self-image, and spirituality. Experience of moral distress also influences attitudes toward the nurse's execution of personal advance directives and participation in blood donation and organ donation. Critical care nurses commonly encounter situations that are associated with high levels of moral distress and the impact of this distress has implications that extend well beyond job satisfaction and retention. Thus, it is critical that strategies to mitigate moral distress in nurses should be developed (Elpern, Covert, & Kleinpell, 2005).

Recognizing moral distress can lead to a significant shift in the way moral choices are perceived and the moral context of practice understood. Nurses use a variety of coping mechanisms to deal with moral distress. They might choose to remain silent, act secretly, and/or use their work with patients and families to sustain them (Austin et al., 2005). As was the case with Kate, some nurses decide to take a stance and act on it. Although she sought support from colleagues, as many nurses do, she found little support in the environment in which she worked. In situations where patients request assistance in dying, the nurse participants in one study responded by various ways. While some nurses refused assistance, or acted by administering palliative drugs that might secondarily hasten dying, other nurses choose to tacitly permit assisted suicide by not interfering with patient or family plans to hasten death. Still others actively provided direct assistance in dying. The various choices these nurses made were context driven and secrecy and collusion were common. Most nurses in this study struggled to balance the moral and legal aspects of helping patients die well. Regardless of their decisions and actions, nurses who believed they had hastened death described feelings of guilt and moral distress (Schwarz, 2004).

Given the complexities of the health care system today, and the profound and lingering effects of choosing to assist individuals in dying, whether tacitly or actively, it is important to critically examine these issues and provide opportunities for nurses working with the terminally ill to meet with supportive colleagues. By providing a safe environment within which nurses can share their experiences with troubling cases and of moral conflict, lasting effects of moral distress such as burnout and substance abuse might be avoided.

Spirituality, Nursing, and Decision-Making: Where to Go from Here?

Thus far, this chapter has examined the influence of morals, values, and spirituality on decision-making from the perspectives of patients, families, and health professionals. A series of case studies were used to help explore the complexities and often paradoxical links between religious belief and end-of-life decision-making. What is clear from these case studies is that although groups of people might share a common set of religious tenets and beliefs, each individual's perceptions of the meaning of these beliefs and how they should be acted on differs considerably within the group. Spiritual faith is not static and it changes in the context of time and experience. Moreover, one's spirituality is often influenced by a dynamic interaction among social, cultural, physical, and psychological factors that shade one's perception and interpretation of life events. For example, even though an individual might execute an advance directive when they are healthy, in the face of acute illness, they might well change their mind and request aggressive therapies that might or might not be appropriate. Even those who have deep spiritual faith can be fearful in the face of death.

There is a growing body of literature in the role of religion and spirituality in individual and familial end-of-life decision-making. This literature reveals a dissonance between the needs of medical institutions, health professionals, and the critically ill. In the 1970s, the ethics literature was full of compelling testimonials of those who believed their loved ones were terminally ill. In one case, the parents of a premature infant wrote that their dying infant was "entrapped in an intensive care unit where the machinery is [was] more sophisticated than the code of law and ethics governing its use" (Stinson & Stinson, 1981, p. 5). More currently, as Kirschbaum (1996) points out, the ethics literature "has swung to describe parents' demands for futile treatment as autonomy gone wild" (p. 51). There is ample evidence of the increasing conflict between religious convictions of patients and their families and professional clinical decision-making (Brett & Jersild, 2003). Although the literature on interventions to help patients' professionals and families to reframe their convictions in ways that might be mutually beneficial is sparse, it does exist (Brett & Jersild, 2003; Okon, 2005). As noted in the neonatal intensive care case study, there were things that the staff could have done to promote a more positive outcome for the parents. While the loss of an infant is devastating, if the staff understood the complexities of the parents' reactions, listened carefully to their concerns, and viewed the situation from their perspectives, the results might have been quite different.

Okon (2005) provides a comprehensive review of the spiritual aspects of palliative care and details the various instruments used in clinical research, assessment tools, approaches to conducting spiritual histories from religious and existential perspectives, and effective communication techniques. Regardless of the tools that are used as a basis for assessment and discussion, a few principles should be considered.

Several of the case studies presented in this chapter demonstrate how difficult situations can be managed in a positive manner. In Hannah's case, the hospice staff had an open and honest discussion about Tina's beliefs and her coworkers' concerns. In doing so, they identified a potential source of conflict and developed a plan to help Hannah's parents during a difficult time. Although Hannah's parents came to a decision that was consistent with Tina's beliefs, they did so for very different reasons. The process by which these issues were raised and discussed in this case is consistent with recommendations in much of the literature on moral distress in nurses. The hospice team effectively created a culture of caring that valued honesty and respected autonomy while maintaining their obligations to Hannah's family.

Although there is debate over the appropriate role for nurses in providing spiritual care for their patients (van Leeuwen et al., 2006) it is clear that nurses' spiritual and religious beliefs shape their interactions with their colleagues and patients. While some nurses are comfortable discussing spiritual concerns with patients and their families when they arise, many nurses are not. The Working Group on Religious and Spiritual Issues at the End of Life has set guidelines in regard to health professionals attending to the spiritual needs of patients. The guidelines encourage listening carefully to patients and to show respect for their views but avoid theological discussions unless having the requisite training to do so and this is requested by the patient. The guidelines also suggest that appropriate professional resources should be used to support the patient, such as a referral to a chaplain or as in Mary and Leonard's case, the patient's minister or parish nurse.

Conclusion

The case studies in this chapter highlight real-life exemplars of the interrelationships between spirituality beliefs and practices and clinical decision-making. When confronted with issues of living and dying, each person comes with their unique perspective and handles these issues in their own time and in their own way. Although there are guides available to assist nurses, it is important to remember this when working with patients and their families. Nurses can best support each other, patients, and their families if they reflect on their own spirituality while listening carefully and respecting the views of others.

References

Albrecht, S. A., Reynolds, M. D., Cornelius, M. D., Heidinger, J., & Armfield, C. (2002). Connectedness of pregnant adolescents who smoke. *Journal of Child & Adolescent Psychiatric Nursing*, 15(1), 16–23.

Allen, W. (2005). Erring too far on the side of life: Deja vu all over again in the Schiavo saga. *Stetson Law Review*, 35(1), 123–145.

Antonovsky, A. (1979). *Health, stress, and coping*. San Francisco, CA: Jossey Bass, Inc.

Amenta, M. O. R. (1984). Traits of hospice nurses compared with those who work in traditional setting. *Journal of Clinical Psychology*, 40(2), 414–420.

Annas, G. J. (2005). "I want to live": Medicine betrayed by ideology in the political debate over Terri Schiavo. *Stetson Law Review*, 35(1), 49–80.

Austin, W., Rankel, M., Kagan, L., Bergum, V., & Lemermeyer, G. (2005). To stay or to go, to speak or stay silent, to act or not to act: Moral distress as experienced by psychologists. *Ethics & Behavior*, 15(3), 197–212.

Bergan, A. E., & Jensen, J. P. (1990). Religiosity of psychotherapists: A national survey. *Psychotherapy*, 27, 3–7.

Brett, A., & Jersild, P. (2003). "Inappropriate" treatment near the end of life: Conflict between religious convictions and clinical judgment. *Archives of Internal Medicine*, 163, 1645–1649.

Buck, J. (2004). Home health versus home hospice: Cooperation, competition and co-optation. *Nursing History Review*, 12, 25–46.

Buck, J. (2005). *Rights of passage: Reforming care for the dying, 1965–1986*. Charlottesville: University of Virginia.

Buck, J. (2006). "Manna from heaven": Religion, nursing, and the modern hospice concept. *Windows in Time*, 14(1), 6–9.

Buck, J. (2007). Reweaving a tapestry of care: Nursing, religion and the meaning of hospice, 1945–1978. *Nursing History Review*, 15, 113–145.

Buhler-Wilkerson, K. (2001). *No place like home: A history of nursing & home care in the United States*. Baltimore, MD: The Johns Hopkins University Press.

Caralis, P., Davis, B., Wright, K., & Marcial, E. (1993). The influence of ethnicity and race on attitudes toward advance directives, life-prolonging treatments, and euthanasia. *The Journal of Clinical Ethics*, 4, 155–165.

Cassel, E. (1974). Death in a technological society. In P. Steifels & R. Veatch (Eds.), *The Hastings Center Report: Death inside out*. New York: Harper and Row.

Cerminara, K. L. (2005). Tracking the storm: The far-reaching power of the forces propelling the Schiavo cases. *Stetson Law Review*, 35(1), 147–178.

Clark, D. (1997, August 20–26). Someone to watch over me . . . Cicely Saunders. *Nursing Times*, 93(34), 50–52.

Clark, D. (1998). Originating a movement: Cicely Saunders and the development of St. Christopher's Hospice, 1957–1967. *Mortality*, 3(1), 43–63.

Cohen, L. M. (2006). Shattering the consensus on end-of-life care: Was the Schiavo case palliative medicine's Humpty Dumpty? *Palliative & Supportive Care*, 4(2), 113–116.

Corley, M. C., Minick, P., Elswick, R. K., & Jacobs, M. (2005). Nurse moral distress and ethical work environment. *Nursing Ethics,* 12(4), 381–390.

Cotton, S., Larkin, E., Hoopes, A., Cromer, B. A., & Rosenthal, S. L. (2005). The impact of adolescent spirituality on depressive symptoms and health risk behaviors. *Journal of Adolescent Health,* 36(6), 472–480.

Daugherty, C., Fitchett, G., Murphy, P., Peterman, A., Banik, D., Hlubocky, F., et al. (2004). Trusting God and medicine: Spirituality in advanced cancer patients volunteering for clinical trials of experimental agents. *Psycho-Oncology,* 14, 135–146.

du Boulay, S. (1984). *Cicely Saunders, founder of the modern hospice movement.* New York: Amaryllis Press.

Duff, R., & Hollingshead, A. (1968). *Sickness and society.* New York: Harper & Row.

Ellison, C. G., & Levin, J. S. (1998). The religion-health connection: Evidence, theory, and future directions. *Health Education Behavior,* 25, 700–720.

Elpern, E. H., Covert, B., & Kleinpell, R. (2005). Moral distress of staff nurses in a medical intensive care unit. *American Journal of Critical Care,* 14(6), 523–530.

Feher, S., & Maly, R. (1999). Coping with breast cancer in later life: The role of religious faith. *Psycho-Oncology,* 8, 408–416.

Fenton, M. (1988). Moral distress in clinical practice: Implications for the nurse administrator. *Canadian Journal of Nursing Administration,* 1, 8–11.

Ferrell, B. R. (2006). Journal club. Understanding the moral distress of nurses witnessing medically futile care. *Oncology Nursing Forum,* 33(5), 922–930.

Filene, P. (1998). *In the arms of others: A cultural history of the right to die in America.* Chicago: Ivan Dee.

Fins, J. J. (2006). Affirming the right to care, preserving the right to die: Disorders of consciousness and neuroethics after Schiavo. *Palliative & Supportive Care,* 4(2), 169–178.

Gallup, G., & Lindsay, D. (1999). *Surveying the religious landscape: Trends in U.S. beliefs.* Harrisburg, PA: Morehouse Publishing.

Ganzini, L. (2006). Artificial nutrition and hydration at the end of life: Ethics and evidence. *Palliative & Supportive Care,* 4(2), 135–143.

Garrett, J., Harris, R., Norburn, J., Patrick, D., & Danis, M. (1993). Life-sustaining treatments during terminal illness: Who wants what? *Journal of General Internal Medicine,* 8, 361–368.

Gee, R. (2006). Plan B, reproductive rights, and physician activism. *New England Journal of Medicine,* 355(1), 4–5.

Glaser, B., & Strauss, A. (1965). *Awareness of dying.* Chicago: Aldine Publishing Company.

Glaser, B., & Strauss, A. (1968). *Time for dying.* Chicago: Aldine Press.

Humphrey, D., & Wickett, A. (1986). *The Right to Die: Understanding Euthanasia* (New York: Harper & Row).

Humphreys, C. (2001). "Waiting for the last summons": The establishment of the first hospices in England, 1878–1914. *Mortality,* 6(2), 146–166.

Hutchinson, C. (1998). Phase I trials in cancer patients: Participants' perceptions. *European Journal of Cancer Care,* 7, 15–22.

Jackson, F., Schim, S., & Seely, S. (2000). Barriers to hospice care for African Americans: Problems and solutions. *Journal of Hospice and Palliative Nursing, 2,* 65–72.

Jenkins, R. A., & Pargament, K. (1995). Religion and spirituality as resources for coping with cancer. *Journal of Psychosocial Oncology, 13,* 51–74.

Johnson, K., Elbert-Avila, K., & Tulsky, J. (2005). The influence of spiritual beliefs and practices in the treatment preferences of African Americans: A review of the literature. *Journal of the American Geriatrics Society, 53,* 711–719.

Johnson, M. (2006). Terri Schiavo: A disability rights case. *Death Studies,* 30(2), 163–176.

Kirschbaum, M. S. (2006). Life support decisions for children: What do parents value? *Advances in Nursing Science, 19*(1), 51–71.

Koenig, H. (2004). Religion, spirituality, and medicine: Research findings and implications for clinical practice. *Southern Medical Journal, 97*(12), 1194–2000.

Krisman-Scott, M. A. (2001). Origins of hospice in the United States: The care of the dying, 1945–1975. *Journal of Hospice and Palliative Nursing, 5*(4), 205–212.

Kübler-Ross, E. (1969). *On death and dying.* New York: Macmillan House.

Leblanc, A. J., Driscoll, A. K., & Pearlin, L. I. (2004). Religiosity and the expansion of caregiver stress. *Aging & Mental Health, 8*(5), 410–421.

Lehrer, J. A., Shrier, L. A., Gortmaker, S., & Buka, S. (2006). Depressive symptoms as a longitudinal predictor of sexual risk behaviors among U.S. middle and high school students. *Pediatrics, 118*(1), 189–200.

Marks, T. C. (2005). A dissenting opinion, *Bush v. Schiavo,* 885 So. 2d 321 (Fla. 2004). *Stetson Law Review, 35*(1), 195–205.

Matzo, M. L. (1996). Registered nurses' attitudes toward and practices of assisted suicide and patient-requested euthanasia. Unpublished doctoral dissertation. University of Massachusetts at Boston.

McSherry, W., & Cash, K. (2004). The language of spirituality: An emerging taxonomy. *International Journal of Nursing Studies, 41,* 151–161.

Meltzer, L. S., & Huckabay, L. M. (2004). Critical care nurses' perceptions of futile care and its effect on burnout. *American Journal of Critical Care, 13*(3), 202–208.

Merriam-Webster's. (2003). Merriam-Webster's collegiate dictionary, 11th ed. Springfield, MA: Merriam-Webster Inc.

Nathaniel, A. (2002). Moral distress among nurses. *The American Nurses Association Ethics and Human Rights Issues Update, 1*(3), 1–8.

O'Brien, M. E. (1999). *Spirituality in nursing: Standing on holy ground.* London: Jones and Bartlett Publishers International.

Okon, T. (2005). Spiritual, religious, and existential aspects of palliative care. *Journal of Palliative Medicine, 8*(2), 392–419.

Pannier, E. (1980). *The hospice caregiver: A qualitative study.* Evanston, IL: Northwestern University.

Pargament, K. L., Van Haitsma, K. S., & Ensing, D. S. (1995). Religion in coping. In M. A. Kimble, S. H. McFadden, J. W. Ellor, & J. J. Seeber (Eds.), *Aging, spirituality, and religion: A handbook* (pp. 47–49). Minneapolis, MN: Fortress Press.

Paris, J. J. (2006). Terri Schiavo and the use of artificial nutrition and fluids: Insights from the Catholic tradition on end-of-life care. *Palliative & Supportive Care,* 4(2), 117–120.

Perry, J. E. (2006). Biblical biopolitics: Judicial process, religious rhetoric, Terri Schiavo and beyond. *Health Matrix,* 16(2), 553–630.

Post-White, J., Ceronsky, C., Kreitzer, M., Nickelson, K., Drew, D., Mackey, K. W., et al. (1996). Hope, spirituality, sense of coherence, and quality of life in patients with cancer. *Oncology Nursing Forum,* 23(10), 1571–1579.

Quint, J. (1967). *The nurse and the dying patient.* New York: The Macmillan Company.

Reesek, D. J., Ahren, R. E., & Nair, S. (1999). Hospice access and use by African Americans: Addressing cultural and institutional barriers through participatory action research. *Social Work,* 44, 549–559.

Roscoe, L. A., Osman, H., & Haley, W. E. (2006). Implications of the Schiavo case for understanding family caregiving issues at the end of life. *Death Studies,* 30(2), 149–161.

Schwartz, M., Hughes, C., Roth, J., Main, D., Peshkin, B., Isaacs, C., et al. (2000). Spiritual faith and genetic testing decisions among high-risk breast cancer probands. *Cancer Epidemiology, Biomarkers and Prevention,* 9, 381–385.

Schwarz, J. (2004). Responding to persistent requests for assistance in dying: A phenomenological inquiry. *International Journal of Palliative Nursing,* 10(5), 225–235.

Schwarz, J., & Coyle, N. (2006). Can we know what Terri Schiavo would have wanted? *Palliative & Supportive Care,* 4(2), 129–133.

Shahabi, L., Powell, L., Musick, M., Pargament, K., Thoresen, C., & Williams, D. (2002). Correlates of self-perceptions of spirituality in American adults. *Annals of Behavioral Medicine,* 24, 59–68.

Shapiro, J., Radecki, S., Charchian, A. S., & Josephson, V. (1999). Sexual behavior and AIDS-related knowledge among community college students in Orange County, California. *Journal of Community Health,* 24(1), 29–43.

Shelley, J., & Miller, A. B. (1999). *Called to care: A Christian theology of nursing.* Downers Grove, IL: InterVarsity Press.

Siebold, C. (1992). *The hospice movement: Easing death's pain.* New York: Twayne Publishers.

Smith, S., & Nickel, D. (1999). From home to hospital: Parallels in birthing and dying in twentieth-century Canada. *Canadian Bulletin of Medical History,* 16(1), 49–64.

Strawbridge, W. J., Shema, S. J., Cohen, R. D., Roberts, R. E., & Kaplan, G. A. (1998). Religiosity buffers effects of some stressors on depression but exacerbates others. *Journals of Gerontology Series B-Psychological Sciences & Social Sciences,* 53(3), S118–S126.

Stinson, R., & Stinson, P. (1981). On the death of a baby. *Journal of Medical Ethics,* 7, 5–18.

Stutts, A., & Schloemann, J. (2002). Life-sustaining support: Ethical, cultural and spiritual conflicts, Part II: Staff support—A neonatal case study. *Neonatal Network,* 21(4), 27–34.

Sudnow, D. (1967). *Passing on: The social organization of dying.* Upper Saddle River, NJ: Prentice Hall.

Tanyi, R. (2002). Toward clarification of the meaning of spirituality. *Journal of Advanced Nursing, 39*(5), 500–509.

Taylor, E. J. (2006). Prevalence and associated factors of spiritual needs among patients with cancer and family caregivers. *Oncology Nursing Forum, 33*(4), 729–735.

True, G., Phipps, E., Braitman, L., Harralson, T., Harris, D., & Tester, W. (2005). Treatment preferences and advance care planning at end of life: The role of ethnicity and spiritual coping in cancer patients. *Annals of Behavioral Medicine, 30*(2), 174–179.

van Leeuwen, R., Tiesinga, L., Post, D., & Jochemsen, H. (2006). Spiritual care: Implications for nurses' professional responsibility. *Journal of Clinical Nursing, 15*(7), 875–884.

Walsh, J. (1929). *The history of nursing.* New York: PJ Kennedy and Sons.

Webb, M. (1997). *The good death: The new American search to reshape the end of life.* New York: Bantam Books.

Wolfson, J. (2005). The rule in Terri's case: An essay on the public death of Theresa Marie Schiavo. *Stetson Law Review, 35*(1), 39–47.

Wortham, C. B. (1989). *An investigation of the influence of religiosity on the ease with which nurses respond to death and dying situations.* Atlanta, GA: Emory University.

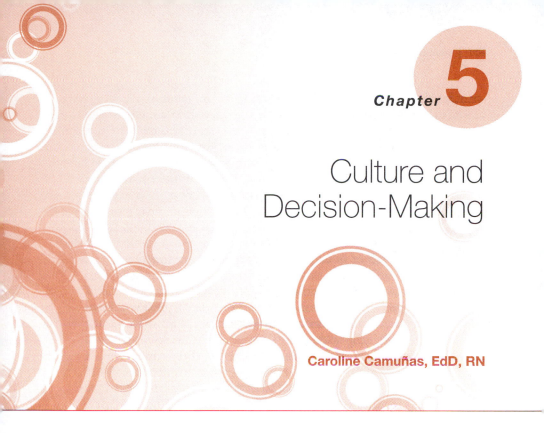

Chapter 5

Culture and Decision-Making

Caroline Camuñas, EdD, RN

D ecision-making is a complex process. It involves gathering and making sense of a great deal of information; culture makes up a large part of that information. Culture has an important impact on the quality of our decision-makings and their outcomes. Astute, knowledgeable, considered application of culture theory is essential for effective, appropriate decision-makings. As nurses, we have learned the importance of making such on-target decision-makings to improve patient care, work relationships, and myriad outcomes.

Case Study

Several years ago, I volunteered and taught nursing in Vietnam with Health Volunteers Overseas (HVO). At the end of a meeting at the ministry of health in Hanoi, one of the women walked me to the front gate of the ministry compound; the distance was about a city block. Just

71

after we left the building, Dinh took my hand and held it until we reached the taxi at the curb. Now, I knew that same sex friends often hold hands in Vietnam. I managed to hold Dinh's hand for the journey, but my immediate reaction was to extricate my hand: I had to reassure and make myself keep holding her hand. It was not easy. I am sure that on earlier occasions in Vietnam, I did not walk holding hands; I have seen countless colleagues drop hands right away, even when they know that it is the custom. This is just an example of taken-for-granted behavior of those of one culture being unacceptable by those of another. The gesture is one of friendship and can be as offensive and rejected by the receiver as the rejection can be felt as hurtful and rude by the handholder. A seemingly small, insignificant culture act can cause great misunderstanding and deepen culture shock.

The Vietnamese with whom we worked a great deal knew that we were not comfortable holding hands. By the same token, those of us who spent time with them learned and were eventually able to hold hands. Culture is adaptable and changes all the time. Traditionally the teacher is accorded high status and students are there to listen and learn, not to question. Students are seated in neat rows. Being American, the volunteers who went to teach faculty rearranged the classroom in a circle. The Vietnamese faculty were game and adapted to, and learned, and then over time adopted the U.S. teaching strategies. Those making decision-makings must consider culture carefully, seriously, and competently. Such decision-makings require sensitivity, understanding your relationship and your responsibility, and your trust and your respect for the autonomy of others.

Culture

Culture has various definitions. The discipline of philosophy defines culture as the way of life of a people, including their attitudes, values, beliefs, arts, sciences, modes of perception, and habits of thought and activity. Cultural features of forms of life are learned but are often too pervasive to be readily noticed from within (Blackburn, 1996). Anthropologist Margaret Meade understood culture to mean "the systematic body of learned behavior which is transmitted from parents to children (Macklin, 1999, p. 6). For nursing, Purnell and Paulanka (1998) define culture as the totality of socially transmitted behavioral patterns, arts, beliefs, values, customs, life ways, and all other products of human work and thought characteristics of a population of people that guide their worldview and decision-making. Yet another definition of culture important to nurses is one used by business. Organizational culture is important in the business world and is defined as the pattern of role-related beliefs, values, and expectations that are shared by members of an organization. These patterns produce the rules and norms of behavior that have a powerful influence on individual and group behavior within the organization. Role-related values of a person are made of the individual's personal values and organizational values. (See **Table 5-1**.)

Organizational culture is important to nurses and nursing because it has an important impact on all individuals, whether patients, nurses, or other employees. There is a direct link between a multifaceted bottom line and the prevalent culture. An important example is the culture shock nurses suffer when their values conflict with that of the organization (Kramer, 1974; Kramer & Schmalenberg, 1977). Culture shock is turmoil or a disturbance of mental equilibrium that includes feelings of helplessness, powerlessness, frustration, and dissatisfaction when a new culture or subculture is encountered. Attempts are made to understand and effectively adapt to the different group or practice. It also can be experienced in one's own culture when a new or novel event or circumstance takes place. Any and all who come in contact with the health care system can experience culture shock.

Cultural diversity is exemplified by immigrant or minority families and groups and includes individual families who have their own blend of group and personal characteristics. Within each family, individuals have their own beliefs, hopes, strengths, weaknesses, limitations, and goals; special group and personal characteristics developed over generations through shared history. Ignoring important aspects of cultural

Table 5-1

Organizational Culture: Shared Values

Personal Values	Role-Related Values	Organizational Values
Ambition	Ambition	Leadership in care and science
Beneficence	Beneficence	Beneficence; excellence
Compassion	Compassion	Service quality
Courage	Patient satisfaction	Patient satisfaction
Excellence	Excellence	Improved decision-making
Fairness, justice	Competence	Internal competition
Family	Ingenuity, creativity	External competition
Honesty, truth	Honesty, truth	Honesty, truth
Independence	Resourcefulness	Innovation
Integrity	Integrity	Efficiency & cost control
Loyalty	Shared goals	Shared goals
Respect for autonomy	Respect for autonomy	Respect for employee and patient autonomy
Responsibility	Responsibility	Responsibility
Nonmaleficence	Nonmaleficence	Nonmaleficence

Source: Adapted from Dickson, P. R. (1994). The shared values that make an organizational culture. In *Marketing management.* New York: Dryden Press.

diversity have led to major disparities in health care. The literature is replete with research evidence that demonstrates prevalent race and gender discrimination in health care allocation (Bach, Pham, Schrag, Tate, & Hargraves, 2004; Bloche, 2004; Haiman et al., 2006; Smedley, Stith, & Nelson, 2003; Steinbrook, 2004). Such evidence shows that culture often has been absent from decision-making regarding the planning, implementation, and evaluation of the health care system.

Health care providers increasingly encounter persons from diverse cultures. The population of the United States is becoming more diverse; while all minority groups are growing, some, such as Hispanics are growing faster than others. It is not too difficult to foresee a future where every group is a minority. As minority groups grow, that growth is not reflected in the nursing work force (see **Table 5-2**). This may well portend more difficulties in providing appropriate, effective care.

Leininger and McFarland (2006) affirm that nursing is a unique caring profession that serves others around the world, and that nursing is affected by ethnohistory, culture, social structures, and environmental factors in varied areas and by the different needs of people. In order to practice, nurses must include culture, religion, spirituality, social change, and multiple other facets that influence health and well-being. This knowledge is necessary to help people with their diverse care needs.

Analysis of these factors or influencers led Leininger to identify three main actions and decision-making guides to provide safe, culturally congruent, and meaningful health care to those of different cultures. These guides were: (1) culture care preservation and/or maintenance, (2) culture care accommodation and/or negotiation, and (3) culture care repat-

Table 5-2

Diversity: United States Population and Nurse Population

	Total Population	Percent	Nurses	Percent
USA	281,421,906	100	2,696,540	100
White	211,460,626	75.1	2,333,896	86.6
Black	34,658,190	12.3	133,041	4.9
Hispanic	35,305,818	12.5	54,861	2.0
Asian	10,242,998	3.6	93,415	3.5
American Indian Alaska Native	2,475,956	0.88	13,040	0.5
Native Hawaiian Pacific Islander	398,835	0.14	6,475	0.2
Other	15,359,073	5.5	61,812	2.3

Note: Total population percentage more than 100% (as Hispanic) may include other ethnic groups.
Source: US Census Bureau, Census 2000, Summary File 1 and USDHHS, Health Resource and Service Administration, Bureau of Health Professions, Division of Nursing, March 2000.

terning and/or restructuring. Reviewing the faculty response to teaching methods in the case study, it is easy to see that it corresponds to this guide.

Patterns of Knowing

Culture is a part of the body of knowledge that nurses use. Carper, in her seminal study (1978), identified that the patterns, forms, and structures of knowledge nurses use in practice consist of (1) empirics, (2) esthetics, (3) personal knowledge, and (4) ethics or moral knowledge. *Empirics*, or the science of nursing, is concerned with describing, explaining, and predicting phenomena. *Esthetics*, or the art of nursing, is the expressive and perceptive aspect of nursing that is little understood. *Personal knowledge* ". . . is concerned with the knowing, encountering, and actualizing of the concrete, individual self" (p.18). *Ethics* is philosophy regarding morality and focuses on right and wrong, good and bad; it is about the "why?" of morality. Philosophy attempts to explicate or answer why this is right or wrong, good or bad.

Science is the method through which knowledge of human beings and the world is organized. Factors such as intuition, experience, and good judgment contribute to new knowledge in science (Chernow & Vallasi, 1993, p. 2452). Rogers (1988) asserted that it is through "the imaginative and creative use of knowledge that nurses can know and understand the health care needs of people" (p. 10). Knowledge development and research are generally embedded in cultural values and perspectives. We study what is important to us; what is important to us generally has a cultural base (Ketefian & Redman, 1977).

Johnson (1994), in a dialectical study, identified five distinct conceptualizations that can be identified as art. These distinct conceptualizations are:

1. Grasping meaning in patient encounters
2. Establishing a meaningful connection with the patient
3. Performing nursing activities skillfully
4. Determining an appropriate course of action rationally
5. Conducting one's nursing practice ethically

Understanding meaning is essential; attention must be paid to experience. Lack of attention to experience is a disservice to patients and can put them at risk. Chinn and Kramer (1991) understand esthetic knowing as what makes possible what to do with the moment, instantly, without conscious deliberation (p. 10).

Carper (1978) acknowledged that personal knowledge is the "most problematic, the most difficult to master and to teach" (p.18). It is also essential to understanding the person (patient) before you. Interpersonal relationships, interactions, and transactions are intrinsic to nursing.

This process is of primary concern in a healing relationship. Personal knowing requires that you are in relationship with the human being as a person. There must be an openness, a freedom from categories, classifications, and pigeonholes. We must be in a relationship that is not generalized by beliefs, concepts, expectations, and stereotypes. In doing so, we have to be willing and able to accept ambiguity, vagueness, and discrepancy of others and ourselves.

Ethics is the fourth pattern of knowing identified by Carper (1978). Moral discomfort and moral dilemmas arise in situations of uncertainty and ambiguity. Nonmaleficence and beneficence are principles basic to nursing practice along with principles of respect for autonomy and justice. Beyond principles is care and caring or care-based ethics, which is another approach to understanding moral life. Care has developed as a theory of ethics that is important in private life (family and friends) as well as in public life (law, medical, and nursing practice, politics, the organization of society, war, and international relations). Care-based ethics is concerned with how we do what we do.

Care and Caring

In health care, care is talked about in several ways. First, care is understood as physical as in taking care of or doing something for another; it is an activity. The second sense of care is to use caution or to be careful to do something correctly in order to avoid accident, injury, or hurt. These two meanings have to do with the cognitive and psychomotor domains in education. The third sense of care deals with emotion and attitude and falls within the affective domain. Care-based ethics is concerned with the third meaning: the affective meaning, of care and caring and how nurses enrich patient care and their profession by developing and practicing care and caring.

Beauchamp and Childress (2001) and Barnum (1998) assert that the expression of caring makes a critical difference. Professional skill is effectively enhanced with caring. When caring is absent, nurses can fail patients in important ways. Emotional engagement and communication are important parts of human relationships in general and health care in particular. However, caring is not sufficient; cognitive and psychomotor skills are essential. Ideas central to care are: (1) mutual interdependence, (2) emotional response, (3) relationship, (4) responsibility, (5) particularity, (6) interrelationship, (7) engagement, and (8) attentive discernment. See **Table 5-3** for major features of care-based ethics.

Care involves a wide range of perceptual, imaginative, emotional, and expressive capacities. Emotions are important to discernment or development of acute judgment and understanding the conditions of others. We often discern the condition of others through our emotions. For

---

Table 5-3

Major Features of Care-Based Ethics

---

1. Attends to and meets the needs of the particular others with whom we are in relationship and for whom we take responsibility.

2. Tries to understand what morality would recommend and what it would be morally best for us to do and to be; emotion is valued and has a moral role.

3. Rejects impartiality seen in the dominant moral theories. Respects rather than removes itself from the claims of particular others with whom we share actual relationships; values engagement.

4. Reconceptualizes mutual interrelationship as feeling for and being immersed in the other, so that the moral response is attentive discernment rather than detached respect for rights.

5. Conceives of persons as relational and who remain so.

6. Involves insight and understanding of circumstances, needs, and feelings that includes or requires a cognitive dimension.

---

example, my own capacity for humiliation can tune me into the fact that a course of treatment is humiliating and debilitating for a patient rather than just uncomfortable or mildly embarrassing. An important question concerns what traits and capacities ought I develop as a person who must engage with and care for others.

Unknowing

These fundamental patterns are important in the consideration of culture and decision-making yet, they are not the whole of knowing. Munhall (1993) identified and explicated how unknowing is important for nurses because it makes them authentically present for the patient. Unknowing is essential to understanding the intersubjective and the perspective. Munhall asserts that it is "essential that we understand our self and our patient to be two distinctive beings, one of whom we do not know" (p. 125). Intersubjectivity is the verbal and nonverbal influence between the organized subjective world of one person and the organized subjective world of another. It is within this intersubjective field that caring, understanding, empathy, conflict, and misunderstandings occur (p. 126). Unknowing is, then, a condition of openness; it allows persons to be. It is "the actual essence of the meaning an experience has for a patient" (p. 128).

Feminist and Womanist

Belenky, Clinchy, Goldberger, and Tarule (1986) identified women's ways of knowing, ways that women nurtured and valued that are powerful but that are looked down upon by the dominant culture. These authors identified that women's voices and ideas are important and valuable. African American women—Banks-Wallace (2000), Boutain (1999), hooks (2000), and Walker (1983), among many others—wrote of womanist knowing. Womanist theory incorporates the theories and practices of feminists and feminism with the traditions of black women. Banks-Wallace (2000) explicates how a womanist epistemological framework can support the development of interventions that assist African American women to include healthful behaviors in their lives. Flaskerud and Nyamathi (2000) compared two conceptual approaches, cultural responsiveness and resource provision, to the inclusion of women and diverse ethnic groups in National Institutes of Health (NIH)–funded research projects. They concluded that cultural responsiveness facilitates participation in research but that provision of resources is important to empower participants to overcome issues of access and burden.

Taylor, Gilligan, and Sullivan (1995) studied culturally diverse urban, poor, and working class children to understand the relationship between risk, resistance, and girls' psychological development and health. They found specific cultural differences that affect girls' coming of age in the United States. The authors also tell a parallel story of African American, Hispanic, and white women who came together to understand their own differences and to learn how to avoid past divisiveness among women. These two findings reveal intergenerational struggle to develop and hold relationships between girls and women and to hold respect for difference.

Feminists reconceptualized traditional notions about the public and the private. The law has not hesitated to intervene into women's private decision-makings concerning reproduction but has been highly reluctant to intrude on men's exercise of coercive power within the "castles" of their homes. Feminism is about equality.

Sociopolitical

White (1995) wrote of *sociopolitical knowing*, which she defined as the context or environment of persons and their interaction. She asserts that this pattern of knowing is essential to understanding the fundamental patterns identified by Carper (1978). White stated that:

> Sociopolitical knowing may be conceptualized as including understandings on two levels: (1) the sociopolitical context of the persons (nurse and patient), and (2) the sociopolitical context as a practice profession, including both society's understanding of nursing and nursing's understanding of society and its politics. (p. 84)

Sociopolitical knowing gives power to patterns of knowing that enable effective policy to be enacted and implemented.

We all make sure we get what we need and want—or, at least we strive mightily to achieve by overcoming obstacles, which are often societal blocks. The women who cannot achieve more because of the glass ceiling are an example. People of color may well know the politics of how to get scarce resources; they often lack the power to succeed. Their uphill battle is often arduous (Wise, 2005).

In-Between and Beyond

Silva, Sorrell, and Sorrell (1995) critiqued Carper's patterns of knowing and identified strengths and weaknesses. Their work grows from a shift in worldview or philosophy. A major contribution made by Carper was that she helped nurses understand that how we come to know is "complex, diverse, ever emerging, and ultimately central to how nurses structure the discipline of nursing" (p. 2). Silva and colleagues advocate for the inclusion of the inexplicable and the unknowable, which relate to the in-between and the beyond. The authors urge nurses to move past epistemological questions to ontological questions that deal with issues of reality, meaning, and being (p. 4). They suggest questions such as "What does my perceptual sensibility to art reveal to me?"; How do I come to know the inexplicable and the unknowable?"; and "What meaning do the inexplicable and unknowable have for me?" (p. 10) The authors maintain that through ontological study, a significant contribution to the foundation of nursing can be made. Such study would broaden and deepen our understanding of culture.

Dialogue

According to Paulo Freire and Donaldo Macedo (1995), dialogue is a way of knowing.

> In order to understand the meaning of dialogical practice, we have to put aside the simplistic understanding of dialogue as a mere technique. Dialogue does not represent a somewhat false path that I attempt to elaborate on and realize in the sense of involving the ingenuity of the other. On the contrary, dialogue characterizes an epistemological relationship. Thus, in this sense, dialogue is a way of knowing and should never be viewed as a mere tactic to involve students in a particular task. We have to make this point very clear. I engage in dialogue not necessarily because I like the other person. I engage in dialogue because I recognize the social and not

merely the individualistic character of the process of knowing. In this sense, dialogue presents itself as an indispensable component of the process of both learning and knowing. (p.10)

Theorizing about the experiences shared in dialogue is part and parcel of Freire's goal learning and knowing (2002). In this way, a curiosity about the object of knowledge has to be always present. Dialogue is not an end; it is a way to better understanding. Dialogue, in this sense, can add immeasurably to understanding of culture.

Judging Other Cultures

Diversity, multiculturalism, and cultural competence are important concepts in nursing today. Emphasis is on accepting and respecting cultural differences, making moral relativism an easy pitfall because there is little to guide professionals in making decisions. Diversity and multicultural populations are increasingly an important aspect of health care in economically developed nations, but there is also migration among developing nations. Hence, the ability to evaluate cultural practices is an important nursing skill worldwide. Multiculturalism in the international context asserts the claim that there are no common moral principles shared by all cultures. Postmodernism asserts a similar claim against all universal standards, both moral and nonmoral.

Around the world, persons, especially women and girls, suffer from physical and emotional oppression in untold numbers. It is hard for Americans to imagine their daily lives. Life expectancy is decreasing dramatically in parts of Africa. There is high infant mortality among girls in some countries and that high rate is linked to discriminatory practices. Malnutrition is prevalent in some countries. There are grave risks for the sexually active. Maternal morbidity and mortality are urgent problems and are recognized by the United Nations and the World Health Organization as an issue of social justice and human rights. These are but a few examples of the outcomes of cultural and political circumstances that constrain persons' lives worldwide.

Important concepts related to culture are cultural imperialism, relativism, and imposition (Purnell, 2001). Often thought of applying to countries, for example, colonization, imperialism is also the installation of policies and practices of one organization to another. Usually the transfer is from the dominant culture to disenfranchised or minority groups. The U.S. government has a history of cultural imperialism. In the early years of the republic, it inflicted grievous harm, even genocide, on Native Americans with forced marches, exposure to smallpox, it stole land and created reservations, and forced their children to attend schools where they learned only the western worldview. The United States is not the only country that has such histories: to whit, the Europeans inflicted genocide on the native peoples of South America and Australia, and dominate groups around the world continue to annihilate minorities. The danger of universal values and standards is the destruction or eradication of traditional cultures worldwide by dominant cultures.

Cultural imposition is the intrusive or disrespectful treatment of individuals and families by dominant culture practices. In health care, policies regarding visiting hours, food service, exclusion of families from plans of care, and informed consent can be seen as imposition. Purnell (2001) advises that nurses must be wary or prudent in expressing their own values. Remember, most nurses in the United States are of European origin and as such are members of the dominant culture.

Cultural relativity and ethical relativism are postmodern theories that assert that cultural practices have traditional roles and can only be evaluated in the context of the particular culture by someone of that culture. This is the defense often used against critical ethical judgments. Anthropologist Mary Catherine Bateson (2000) asserts that we must be able to understand cultural relativity as a principle of method and ethical relativism as philosophy. If ethics are relative to particular cultures or societies, then it is impossible for fundamental human rights to exist. Ruth Macklin (1999), an eminent philosopher and bioethicist, conducted research on cultural relativity and ethical relativism in developing countries throughout the world. Macklin concluded that ethical relativism can be supported for some cultural practices and traditions; for others, it should be rejected as fatal.

What to Do

First, nurses must develop cultural sensitivity. Invest in knowing all that you can; be inquisitive. Looking back on the patterns of knowing, see how you can develop acumen in each area. Science is probably the easiest to accomplish. As nurses and scholars, we are comfortable with science. We have to keep abreast of developments and findings in nursing and other fields. Nurses know how to keep current in their specialization with reading journals, attending conferences, discussions, and so forth.

Esthetics, the second way to know, can decidedly be fun, interesting, and even entertaining. Understanding, knowing through art can be gleaned, for example, through film, fine art, crafts, dance, literature (fiction, nonfiction, and poetry), music and song, theater, museums of all types, and other cultural events.

Literature is an especially rich source for gaining understanding and insight. For instance, female genital mutilation (FGM) is frequently in the news and it is generally laden with emotional response. A good place to start is with the discussion by Nussbaum (1999). Nussbaum, a philosopher, presents a cogent, to-the-point argument with a lot of facts. To understand a piece of the unknowable, turn to Alice Walker's *Possessing the Secret of Joy* (1992). This novel is powerful and goes to the very core of FGM by making real the experience of one woman. Edwidge Danticat probes the issues further with an exploration of how FGM victimizes generations away from the actual cutting experience in *Breath, Eyes, Memory* (1994).

As Carper (1978) stated, personal knowing is the third and most difficult pattern to learn and inculcate into practice. Personal knowing is important in the actualization of an authentic relationship between two persons whose goal is to promote healing. It is learning and developing many characteristics of care-based ethics, which is rooted in receptivity, relatedness, and responsiveness (Noddings, 1984; 2002).

The ethics pattern of knowing has always been important to nurses. Theorists prescribe how nurses ought to act, though ethics may not be intrinsic to the theory but merely superimposed (Barnum, 1998). Educators believe they thread ethics throughout their curricula; generally, they usually fail to achieve this worthy goal. Ethics must be taught so that nurses have the skills needed to recognize and work through situations that have ethics implications. To develop skill in identifying and resolving ethical issues, it is important to have the background knowledge to discuss problems and approaches to resolutions. The dialogue that Freire (2002) speaks is very useful and helpful. It is important to understand that the unexamined is not sufficient to call on when encountering ethical discomfort and dilemmas.

Just as personal knowing is difficult to learn, the pattern of unknowing also is not easy. Munhall states that "a great amount of introspection" is needed (1993, p. 125) and that we "understand our self and our patient to be two distinctive beings, one of whom we do not know" (p. 125). She further asserts that "unknowing is openness" (p. 128).

White (1995) critiqued Carper's 1978 work and added sociopolitical knowing as another pattern. White wrote that sociopolitical knowing moves attention from the "introspective nurse-patient relationship and situates it within the broader context in which nursing and health care take place" (p. 83). To strengthen sociopolitical knowing, become involved in health care politics on community, city, state, and/or national levels. Learn about politics and texts (see Camuñas, 2007; Mason, Leavitt, & Chaffee, 2007, is especially superb). Read newspapers, journals, and editorials; join discussions, committees, and nurses associations; be an active participant. Keep your ears, eyes, and mind open; engage the world.

The ontological in-between and beyond pattern of knowing is seen in phenomenologic and hermeneutic research and in the art, poetry, and narratives created by nurses (Silva et al., 1995). Again, study, read, have dialogues, and engage with art and create art by writing, painting, and so forth. This is important because it assists nurses to provide excellent patient care. The in-betweens and beyonds raise ontological questions about the world; what is meaning, and what is being. Information must not be blindly accepted; it must be critiqued and shared; critical thinking is essential.

All of the patterns of knowing require the dialogue of which Freire speaks. Without this dialogue, learning stands still and our world and our worldviews shrink.

Now that we have discussed patterns of knowing and how to develop those patterns, it must be acknowledged that breaking apart knowing in this way is a means to understand and gain access to the complexity of knowing. As Wilson (1998) eloquently stated, complexity with reductionism makes science and complexity without reductionism makes art. The patterns of knowing are not separate realms; they are extremely complex and interrelated. Just in this brief discussion, each pattern informs the others and ways to one pattern inform other patterns.

Culture and Decision-Making Maker

Culture must be considered in making many decision-makings; critical thinking is essential when making this type of decision-making. Collection of all pertinent data is imperative. Ask questions: Who benefits, who is harmed, what are the benefits, what are the harms. If there are harms associated with the practice or tradition, the decision-making becomes an ethical decision-making. In such a case, certain qualities are demanded of the decision-maker. The decision-maker must be able to recognize ethical issues and to think through the consequences of alternate resolutions. In the example of FGM, the girls and women who are mutilated are harmed. They frequently suffer from life-long chronic illness related to the mutilation such as damaged urinary tracts and infection, difficult and life-threatening labors and deliveries, painful intercourse, and difficult walking and gait, as well as psychological difficulties.

The person who benefits from FGM is the cutter; the mutilator earns a good living and is held in high esteem by the community. Men may think they benefit by the control FGM seems to give them over girls and women. However, in the final analysis, they too are harmed in that they have ill, handicapped, or dead wives and daughters. FGM has a high societal cost. It is interesting and important to note that FGM is illegal in most, if not all, countries in which it is practiced.

Quite tellingly is the fact that in the United Nations' 2000 publication *The World's Women*, FGM is not found in the chapter on health nor is it in the chapter on economics, but, rather, it is in the chapter entitled *Human Rights and Political Decision-Making*. More than half of all girls in some African countries have been subjected to FGM. Unfortunately, the prevalence is not in decline (United Nations, 2000). Amin Maalouf, a Lebanese French author, asserts that many would reject their inherited conceptions of identity, which are kept through force of habit, if they would examine them more closely (2000).

The decision-maker must have the self-confidence to seek out different points of view and then decide what is right at a given time and place in a particular set of relationships and combination of circumstances. We must learn all we can about the situation in order to be able to reach the best decision-making (see **Tables 5-4** and **5-5**). Finally, the decision-maker must be willing to make decisions when all that needs to be known cannot be known and the questions that press for answers have no established and incontrovertible solution.

Table 5-4
Strategies to Facilitate Management of Ethical Decision-Makings
1. Obtain critical facts relevant to the cultural/moral controversy
2. Reach agreement on definition of terms
3. Reach agreement on a common framework of moral principles, concepts, ideas
4. Use examples and counter examples
5. Expose the problems inherent in a line of reasoning

Table 5-5
Important Considerations
1. Medical and nursing data
2. Cultural data
3. Persons or advisors to be consulted in the decision-making process
4. Priority and significance given to values, desires, and opinions of family, significant others, and professionals
5. Documentation of the bioethical/cultural decision-making

Conclusion

We must remember that culture is not static; culture is everchanging. North American cultures are very different at the beginning of the twenty-first century than they were 50 or 100 years ago, or as they were at their foundings. A culture is made up of a plurality of people who have different relationships of power to one another. Some of these relationships are nurturing and sustaining; others may be pathological and detrimental to human flourishing. Nurses must recognize that there are universal principles to protect human flourishing and dignity and we must learn to make decisions that do so.

References

Bach, P. B., Pham, H. H., Schrag, D., Tate, R. C., & Hargraves, J. L. (2004). Primary care physicians who treat blacks and whites. *New England Journal of Medicine, 351*, 575–584.

Banks-Wallace, J. A. (2000). Womanist ways of knowing: Theoretical considerations for research with African American women. *Advances in Nursing Science, 22*(3), 33–45.

Bateson, M. C. (2000). *Full circles, overlapping lives (Culture and generation in transition).* New York: Random House.

Barnum, B. S. (1998). *Nursing theory: Analysis, application, evaluation.* New York: Lippincott.

Beauchamp, T., & Childress, J. (2001). *Principles of biomedical ethics* (5th ed.). New York: Oxford University Press.

Belenky, M. F., Clinchy, B. M. V., Goldberger, N. R., & Tarule, J. M. (1986). *Woman's ways of knowing: The development of self, voice, and mind.* New York: Basic Books.

Blackburn, S. (1996). *Oxford dictionary of philosophy.* New York: Oxford University Press.

Bloche, M. (2004). Health care disparities: Science, politics, and race. *New England Journal of Medicine, 350*, 1568–1570.

Boutain, D. M. (1999). Critical nursing scholarship: Exploring critical social theory with African American studies. *Advances in Nursing Science, 21*(4), 37–47.

Camuñas, C. (2007). Power, politics, and policy. In R. A. P. Jones (Ed.). *Nursing leadership and management: Theory, processes and practice* (pp. 201–220). Philadelphia: F.A. Davis.

Carper, B. (1978). Fundamental patterns of knowing in nursing. *Advances in Nursing, 1*(1), 13–23.

Chernow, B. A., & Vallasi, G. A. (1993). *The Columbia encyclopedia* (5th ed.). New York: Columbia University Press.

Chinn, P. P. L., & Kramer, M. K. (1991). *Theory and nursing: A systematic approach,* 3rd ed. St. Louis, MO: Mosby.

Danticat, E. (1994). *Breath, eyes, memory.* New York: Vintage Books.

Flaskerud, J. H., & Nyamathi, A. M. (2000). Attaining gender and ethic diversity in health intervention research: Cultural responsiveness versus resource provision. *Advances in Nursing Science, 22*(4), 1–15.

Freire, P. (2002). *Pedagogy of the oppressed* (Myra Bergman Ramos, Trans.). New York: Continuum.

Freire, P., & Macedo, D. (1995). A dialogue: Culture, language, and race. *Harvard Educational Review, 65*(3), 379.

Haiman, C. A., Stram, D. O., Wilkins, L. R., Pike, M. C., Kolonel, L. N., et al. (2006). Ethnic and racial differences in smoking-related risk of lung cancer. *New England Journal of Medicine, 354*(4), 333–342.

hooks, b. (2000). *Feminist theory: From margin to center* (2nd ed.). Cambridge, MA: South End Press.

Johnson, J. L. (1994). A dialectical examination of nursing art. *Advances in Nursing Science, 17*(1), 1–14.

Ketefian, S., & Redman, R. W. (1977). Nursing science in the global community. *Image: Journal of Nursing Scholarship, 29,* 11–15.

Kramer, M. (1974). *Reality shock: Why nurses leave nursing.* St. Louis, MO: C.V. Mosby.

Kramer, M., & Schmalenberg, C. (1977). *Path to biculturalism.* Wakefield, MA: Contemporary Publishing.

Leininger, M. M., & McFarland, M. R. (2006). *Culture care, diversity and universality: A worldwide nursing theory* (2nd ed.). Sudbury, MA: Jones & Bartlett.

Macklin, R. (1999). *Against relativism: Cultural diversity and the search for ethical universals in medicine.* New York: Oxford University Press.

Mason, D. J., Leavitt, J. K., & Chaffee, M. W. (Eds.). (2007). *Policy & politics in nursing and health care,* 5th ed. St. Louis, MO: W.B. Saunders.

Maalouf, A. (2000). *In the name of identity: Violence and the need to belong.* New York: Arcade.

Munhall, P. (1993). 'Unknowing': Toward another pattern of knowing in nursing. *Nursing Outlook, 41,* 125–128.

Noddings, N. (1984). *Caring: A feminine approach to ethics & moral education.* Berkeley: University of California Press.

Noddings, N. (2002). *Starting at home: Caring and social policy.* Berkeley: University of California Press.

Nussbaum, M. C. (1999). *Sex and social justice.* New York: Oxford University Press.

Purnell, L. (2001). Cultural competence in a changing health care environment. In N. L. Chaska (Ed.), *The nursing profession: Tomorrow and beyond* (pp. 451–460). Thousand Oaks, CA: Sage.

Purnell, L., & Paulanka, B. J. (1998). *Transcultural health care: A culturally competent approach.* Philadelphia: F.A. Davis.

Rogers, M. E. (1988). Nursing science and art: A prospective. *Nursing Science Quarterly, 1,* 99–102.

Silva, M. C., Sorrell, J. M., & Sorrell, C. D. (1995). From Carper's patterns of knowing to ways of being: An ontological philosophical shift in nursing. *Advances in Nursing Science, 18*(1), 1–13.

Smedley, B. D., Stith, A. Y., & Nelson, A. R. (2003). *Unequal treatment: Confronting racial and ethnic disparities in health care.* Washington, DC: National Academies Press.

Steinbrook, R. (2004). Disparities in health care: From politics to policy. *New England Journal of Medicine, 350,* 1486–1488.

Taylor, J. M. L., Gilligan, C., & Sullivan, A. M. (1995). *Between voice and silence: Women and girls, race and relationship.* Cambridge, MA: Harvard University Press.

United Nations. (2000). *The world's women: Trends and statistics.* New York: Author.

Walker, A. (1983). *In search of our mothers' gardens: Womanist prose.* San Diego, CA: Harcourt Brace Jovanovich.

Walker, A. (1992). *Possessing the secret of joy.* New York: Harcourt Brace Jovanovich.

White, J. (1995). Patterns of knowing: Review, critique, and update. *Advances in Nursing Science, 17*(4), 73–86.

Wilson, E. O. (1998). *Consilience: The unity of knowledge.* New York: Alfred A. Knopf.

Wise, T. (2005). *White like me: Reflections on race from a privileged son.* Brooklyn, NY: Soft Skull Press.

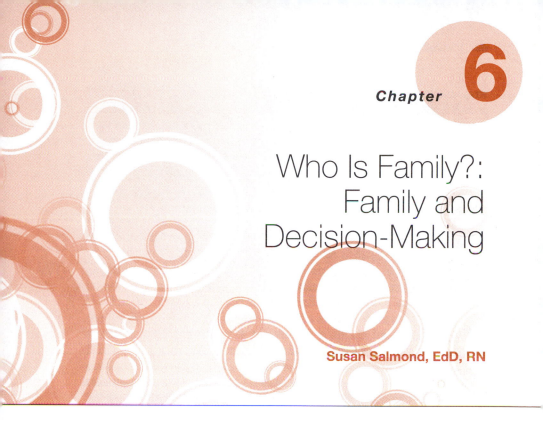

Chapter 6

Who Is Family?: Family and Decision-Making

Susan Salmond, EdD, RN

ealth is created and lived by people within the settings of their everyday life where they learn, work, play, and love (Kickbusch, 1996). Friedman (1998) contends that family is the single most important influencing factor on one's health and that disruptions in health significantly impact the family. Thus, when disease or injury strikes an individual, there is a ripple effect that extends outward from the client to family and friends and into the community itself (Salmond & Spears, 2002). In this ripple, often experienced more like a tidal wave, families are often called upon to make important life decisions on behalf of, or in partnership with the patient, to serve as caregivers, and to advocate the stormy seas of the health care system for their ill relative. Consequently, quality care must be grounded in a family-centered paradigm. Nurses must understand the experience of being a family member of an ill relative, support the family in their own coping, provide information to the family, and involve the family in decision-making responsibilities based on patient preferences and condition. To examine family involvement and decision-making, three case studies are presented in table form throughout the chapter (**Table 6-1**).

Table 6-1

Three Family Case Studies: Part 1

Lisa S., age 33, was a direct admission into the intensive care unit with a diagnosis of status epilepticus. She had been in a neighboring hospital for 2 days and was being transferred to a neurointensive care unit as her condition was not resolving. Lisa was accompanied by her long-term partner, Marie, who was asked to remain in the waiting area. The neurologist contacted Lisa's parents who informed the doctor that Marie knows more about Lisa's recent history and condition. The neurologist provided the parents little information and stated that there was no choice but to induce a coma and that the father would have to consent as Marie was not family. Marie remained in the waiting area for over 2 hours. When she was allowed in to visit, she found Lisa intubated and in a propofol-induced coma. She was angry with the doctors and nurses. She wanted information on the choice of drug used to induce the coma and on the plan to prevent medical complications common while in a coma.

Bill S., age 54, was seen in the emergency room for chest pain. He was accompanied by his wife. EKG was normal, however the blood pressure was high at 190/110 and he was noted to be significantly overweight. A follow-up stress test showed mild ventricular hypertrophy. The nurse practitioner is discussing treatment options with Bill and his wife Nancy. She advises them that the goal is to control the blood pressure better and discusses the pros and cons of increasing medication dosage or control through diet. Given the information, she wants to know what choice seems best to them.

José S., age 84, was admitted into a private room on a medical floor with an inability to bear weight on his right leg. There is significant swelling of the extremity from the ankle to mid-calf. He has a history of advanced prostate cancer with bone metastasis. He is in significant pain and has intermittent disorientation to time, place, and person. He is accompanied by his wife, three nieces, son, and daughter-in-law. His other two sons and their children are on the way. When going in to visit José, the family is stopped and reminded that "this is a hospital and not a social gathering" and "only two people could visit at the same time." Only the wife and son go to visit. The son seeks out the nurse and indicates that his father is not aware of the extent of his condition and he is not to be told. He requests that his brother (the eldest son) be consulted for all decision-making and requests that the family be allowed to come and visit since José is more comfortable when the family is with him. The nurse returns to the nursing station and begins to discuss her concerns with not informing the patient.

Who Is the Family?

Just as the nurse must decide the best approach for dealing with the individual client, so too must the nurse make decisions as to "who" makes up the family and the care that the family needs. Family should be considered as "whoever they say they are." This broad definition of family is consistent with current thinking on relationships within contemporary society. There is no one type of "normal" family, rather there are a variety of family structures: single-parent families, step-families, divorced families, foster families, and extended families which may or may not include fictive kin networks. These many different family types are not better or worse than another and to be therapeutic, the nurse must recognize that many different types of families can work well. Nurses who have a narrower definition of family, such as a traditional nuclear family, may fail to engage the appropriate individuals leaving significant anxiety and frustration as well as health deficits for both the patient and the family.

In the given three case studies, the different types of families include same-sex family, traditional heterosexual, nuclear family; and large extended family. Failure to appropriately engage the "real" family will result in disappointment, anger, resentment, and family and patient stress. These negative emotions were experienced in the first case example by Marie. The physician ignored Lisa's life partner and telephoned Lisa's parents even while Marie remained only doors away in the family waiting area. By the time she got in to see Lisa, she was angry and rightfully so, because she had been left to experience tumultuous fear and no one intervened. Had the nurse advocated for Lisa who could not speak up for herself, the physician would have been informed that the appropriate person to speak with would be Marie and if that was not successful, the nurse could go to the waiting area, provide needed information, and bring Marie to Lisa's bedside. In contrast, the second case study presents a traditional husband and wife and the nurse actively involved the wife. The wife, although anxious, was likely to be relieved to be included in the discussions and therefore could assume an active role in advocating for both Bill and herself. Finally, in the case of José S., the family does not fit the nurse's definition of family and consequently the nurse does not try to intervene to accommodate the extended family or to respectfully interact with the family and negotiate a system for visiting. The nurse, more comfortable with an individualistic style of interaction and decision-making, is uncomfortable with the family-centered approach common to José's culture.

When the health care team engages the patient and the relevant family focusing on both the immediate and longer term health concerns, a "healthy family" concept is promoted and better patient and family outcomes are achieved (Burchard, 2005). This was demonstrated in the case of Bill and Nancy but not with the other case studies (**Table 6-2**).

The Family Role in the Illness Experience

Families influence and are influenced by the health of their members. They assume important roles in health promotion and risk reduction, advocate for the individual experiencing acute illness, and are instrumental as either sources of stress or support as individuals cope with chronic illness. Family members act as buffers for patient anxiety and

Table 6-2

Three Family Case Studies: Part 2

Lisa S. is critically ill and unable to represent herself. In discussions with Marie you find that she has served to monitor Lisa's medication regimen at home in order to help her with compliance. She asks very specific questions demonstrating an in-depth knowledge of the drugs used to manage epilepsy. The nurse apologizes for the wait Marie experienced and verbalizes that it must have been very upsetting to have been excluded from the initial discussion. Marie is invited to remain with Lisa as desired. As care is being given you inquire of Marie to tell you about Lisa as a person. Marie shares stories about Lisa's likes and dislikes, her work and her ambitions, and her general personality. The nurse now has an understanding of Lisa as a person, not just as a young woman in a coma. The nurse explains to Marie Lisa's current condition, the purpose of 24-hour EEG monitoring, and the current treatment plan. Marie inquires as to whether she can stay at Lisa's bedside. She informs the nurse that it would make her more comfortable to be there and talk to Lisa in case she can hear. She also asks if she can be shown how to do passive range of motion to prevent any complications of immobility.

Faced with a serious chronic illness, the treatment goal is blood pressure and weight reduction. In the family conference that is held, Nancy asks many direct questions about the meaning of ventricular hypertrophy and high blood pressure and the consequences if not managed. Bill's initial response was that he would manage the problem by diet. However, Nancy brought forward a different perspective since she was a partner in this discussion. She shared that this was not the first time that Bill had received information about high blood pressure and that past lifestyle changes had been short-lived. It was through this discussion that it was decided that medication would be ordered along with diet changes. It is recognized that Nancy will play a significant role in meal preparation and assisting Bill with goals of weight reduction and increased activity. The nurse offers concrete suggestions of cookbooks that might prove helpful and gives Nancy pamphlets on weight reduction and blood pressure reducing diets.

José's pain is being managed and his intermittent disorientation present on admission is dissipating. After consulting with her colleagues, the nurse has made arrangements for the multiple family members to be present and has requested that they respect the needs of the person in the other bed and not be too noisy. They are sitting quietly when the physician comes in. Speaking directly to José, the physician tells him that he has a tibial fracture and would like to discuss his treatment options. Both José and the family present indicate that they will wait until Juan, the oldest son, arrives before making any decision. The physician leaves but is visibly annoyed with this decision. The nurse asks the family if they have any questions. They indicate they do but would like to talk outside where José cannot hear. You ask permission of José to speak with his family and he says, "Of course—they know what is best." You answer their questions and reassure them that they can wait until the arrival of Juan. The family is upset with the doctor as they have requested in advance a non-disclosure approach. The nurse listens to them. She inquires what they mean by non-disclosure as the physician did not speak of the underlying cause of the fracture (bone metastasis) but spoke of the fracture. The family indicated that they were afraid he would go on to discuss why the fracture occurred. The nurse further inquires about any past confusion episodes and the family provides information on when it has occurred in the past and what they did to manage it and protect him.

serve as valuable resources for patient care (Leske, 2002). In the three case studies, family served critical roles both prior to and after the acute event. Marie served as a control agent, assuring that Lisa took her daily medication regimen as well as serving as a protector for Lisa when she had seizures. Prior to this hypertensive event, Nancy had not been involved in "managing" Bill's health problem; it was his. The nurse recognized that success in meeting health goals required Nancy to be brought into the loop because she would be the person making the meals and assisting to motivate Bill toward his goals. Shared problem-solving between the two would likely have more positive outcomes. José's family shared the responsibility of protectors and caregivers and as is common in many group-oriented cultures, also assumed a decision-making role. By giving the family responsibility for reorienting José and keeping him safe, they felt respected and useful. If the family had not been engaged as occurred in these case studies, quality care would not have been achieved. A family-centered approach to care is emerging in all case studies.

A family-centered paradigm requires the nurse to make the decision to define the "patient" as the actual individual with the disease as well as the family that supports the individual. Research has shown that when care and communication targets the family unit that patients are more satisfied with care, are less anxious, and are more adherent with plans of care (Edwards & Elwyn, 2001).

Gerteis and colleagues published the results of a now-classic study of what matters most to hospitalized patients in the text, *Through the Patient's Eyes* (1993). They identified that the involvement of family and friends was one of eight critical dimensions to care. Patients rely on family members for social and emotional support, to assist with or assume responsibility for problem-solving and decision-making, and to serve as an advocate in assuring quality care and advancing care consistent with the patient's values and preferences. Patients worry about the impact of the illness on the family and when the family is embraced as part of the care unit, then this worry can be minimized.

Among the specialties of pediatrics, palliative care, and oncology, the family-centered paradigm has been actively espoused. Unfortunately for the adult client, the approach is often only individualistic because it is assumed that the individual is the decision-maker and handles his or her own self-management. A family-centered paradigm understands that self-management occurs in the context of the family and the community in which it takes place (Grey, Knafl, & McCorkle, 2006). Failure to incorporate the family knowledge and address family needs will leave significant deficits. Research findings show that health care providers underestimate the extent that families want to be involved and only a minority of patients and family achieve the desired level of involvement

(Bruera, Sweeney, Calder, Palmer, & Benisch-Tolley, 2001; Hack, Degner, Watson, & Sinha, 2005). In the given case studies, the nurses involved the families and from this interaction not only were the families satisfied but the nurse gained "private family" information about the patient that could help guide care. From Marie, the nurse learned of Lisa's love for gospel music; her kind, giving personality; and her mild cognitive deficits that had resulted from previous episodes of status epilepticus. Nancy revealed prior attempts by Bill to manage his high blood pressure and reduce his weight that had been unsuccessful. This information was critical to the ultimate plan of care in this event. José's family shared information about prior disorientation and how the family protected him and reoriented him during these episodes. In these conversations, it was apparent to the nurse that the family was devoted to José and had his best interests at heart which made it easier for the nurse to accept the family as decision-maker rather than the individual.

Another value of the family-centered approach to care is the potential "preventative" role that the model can take. Families are at risk of adverse outcomes as a result of critical or prolonged chronic illness of a loved one. Anxiety, depression, somatization, and symptoms of posttraumatic stress disorder have been found to occur in these families (Cook, 2001). Attending to family needs as part of the care model can help the family to cope with the situation as well as find resources and strategies to support their own needs.

The Impact of Illness on the Family

Fear and anxiety are common emotions for family members as they cope with the uncertainty of illness and their inability to balance change and maintain stability in an environment that is unfamiliar and frequently frightening. Their loved one is at risk for dying or suffering ongoing deficits, and together with unplanned changing family roles, a precarious family situation evolves (Mitchell, Courtney, & Coyer, 2003). Some families may appear overwhelmed with emotions and others may seem confident, knowledgeable, and articulate but they are all dealing with horror and fright and a depth of emotion and turmoil (Taylor, 2006).

When a loved one is hospitalized, they are asked to hand over care to strangers and there are concerns regarding competency and consistency of care. Within what is often an impersonal hospital environment, establishing a respectful relationship between the family and the nurse is crucial. Facilitating open and honest communication and responding to common family concerns are critical components to establishing this relationship. Leske's systematic review (1991) of family needs during acute illness identified three common needs that exist: the need for assurance, the need for proximity, and the need for information. Consciously or unconsciously, nurses control the level of family stress and participation by controlling behavior that impacts these three areas (Corlett & Twycross, 2006).

Assurance comes when the family feels comfortable that the nurse will include the family as partners and are responsive to and understand the patient and the care to be delivered. Begin by communicating an understanding of the stress the family experiences and inquire as to what can be done to assist them. Communicate in a way that maintains hope about the patient's outcome, comfort, and care.

Conveying competence about your ability to provide effective care will assure the family. Share your plan for the shift with the family; let them know what you will be assessing, what treatments you will be giving, and what you will do if the patient's condition changes. After sharing your understanding of the care to be given, ask the family if there are any other needs that have not been considered and that you are available to them.

The need for proximity requires the nurse to negotiate visiting practices for the family. Physical separation is a constant reminder to the family that the illness is accompanied by a danger to the integrity of the family unit and the time in family waiting areas has been found to be exceptionally stressful. Be proactive by promoting family visitation and involvement in the patient's care. This allows the family to remain emotionally close and to give support to the patient. In addition to establishing the mechanism for family access to the patient, it is helpful to identify a primary nursing contact for the family so that consistent communication is facilitated. Additionally, the nurse should establish mechanisms for contacting the family in order to promote family participation and allow for communication with patient changes or when the timing is right within the nurse's shift.

Providing information is key to diminishing some of the anxiety and uncertainty experienced and reciprocal information sharing is part of establishing rapport (Espezel & Canam, 2003). The nurse should explain presenting symptoms and treatments in a meaningful way so that patterns become recognizable and treatment makes sense in light of the symptoms. Information giving must accommodate the family's expected high anxiety: Avoid medical jargon; plan for repetition of information; ask the family what they understand about the situation and provide information based on their understanding and any evident gaps; give opportunity to ask questions and solicit more information; and give emotional support. Supplement conversations or teaching sessions with video tapes, information booklets, or care conferences.

The nurse plays another major role in helping the family to integrate the multiple information input received from an array of providers. Families verbalize frustration with inconsistent and conflicting information as well as receiving only isolated bits of information at a time. The nurse can play a significant role as coordinator for information coming in "system bytes" as one specialist sees a patient and provides information on the kidneys and another specialist sees the patient and provides information on the pulmonary status. Often families interpret specialist information generally. In other words, if the nephrologists says that the kidneys are doing fine, then the family may interpret this as the patient is improving even if the neurological condition is deteriorating. Help the family to see the "big picture" by interpreting the information in light of the patient's overall condition. Do not take away hope but assist the family in understanding the whole.

In all three case studies, the nurses reached out to the family and established a relationship that assisted in allaying some of the family fears and in providing the nurse with information and/or assistance in the care of the client. The nurse apologized to Marie for the long wait and lack of immediate involvement in care and then began to share with her the plan of care. This provided the needed reassurance and allowed Marie to be less defensive and aggressive which had been her initial approach because she had not been involved. Allowing her to stay at her own schedule met the need for proximity and in fact she remained with Lisa about 16 hours per day and was not perceived as a bother but as a support as she performed some basic hygiene care and preventative physical therapy. The nursing staff, now aware of Lisa's likes and dislikes because of their discussions with Marie, encouraged Marie to bring in a tape recorder and gospel music that now played most of the day and evening. In the case of Bill and Nancy, the nurse met the relationship, proximity, and information needs during the acute office visit by including Nancy in the postexam planning and discussion. It was Nancy, not Bill, who provided the nurse with information about past compliance difficulties that were significant in planning what treatment would be prescribed. With José and his family, the nursing staff demonstrated a family-centered approach by respecting the concept of an extended family, negotiating visiting arrangements, and respecting the family's wishes to be the control agent for their father. The nurse provided support to the family when they were upset with the physician's communication and sought information from the family to clarify their meaning of nondisclosure and to gather more information about José's disorientation (**Table 6-3**).

Family Management Styles: One Size Does Not Fit All

One must begin with the premise that there is no "one size fits all" approach for family interaction. Each family presents with their unique family structure, caring styles, family strengths and challenges, and roles they play in the trajectory of the disease. There will be a negoti-

ation process in which it will be determined what the family participation will consist of and what roles the family will have in sharing care
of their sick relative and in the decision-making process.

Table 6-3
Three Family Case Studies: Part 3

Marie is actively involved in the care of Lisa and is most satisfied and relaxed when her information needs are met. The nurse is able to answer questions that Marie has; however, she is requesting more in-depth information about propofol and the nurse gathers this through the hospital intranet. The information is given to Marie. Subsequently the nurse returns and discusses the information that Marie has read and additional questions are answered. She has some concerns with the management plan and the assigned neurologist and is requesting a second opinion from an epileptologist. The nursing staff are supportive of Marie's requests and give her information to help her make decisions about whom to consult. The nursing staff reassures her that her approach is appropriate—that she has Lisa's needs at heart. Marie verbalizes appreciation for the support provided by the nursing staff. She is now verbalizing her concerns about possible functional deficits and complications that may occur. She listens to the nurse's advice and requests that plans be made for getting Lisa out of bed, having a physical therapy consult, and discontinuing the Foley because of the risk for infection.

Nancy and Bill have been included as partners in decision-making. After deciding that medication management would be needed, the pros and cons of different medications are discussed. The couple requests the practitioner to make a decision but want their concerns regarding avoiding medications that would cause sexual dysfunction. Nancy is interested in getting more in-depth information and an education session is established. Bill is not interested in getting more information, He says he knows he has to make changes and will do it. He will rely on his wife for getting the information and helping him to understand. He says that she normally prepares all meals so he will eat whatever she makes for him. He is satisfied with the communication and shared decision-making process.

José's oldest son Juan arrives at the hospital and the family has gone to greet him. The nurse asks José if he has questions about what is happening. He responds, "No, I have no questions." The nurse continues and asks if he would prefer the family to receive the information and he says, "Yes, tell them, my family will take care of everything, they know what is best." The nurse then asks, "Do you want your family to decide with the doctor on your treatment or do you want to be included with your family?" José indicates, "My family will decide and they will take care of me. I am fine." Juan speaks with the nurse and shares that she has spoken with José who has verbalized that his family can be given information and will decide on his treatment. The nurse acknowledges that Juan has been managing José's health concerns for some time and inquires as to the depth of information he prefers to receive. Juan says "I want to know, but I want you to make it understandable—make it simple." The physician tells him that the fracture is due to the spread of the cancer and that he does not recommend surgery but radiation to diminish some of the pain. Juan emphasizes that he wants to make sure that José's pain is not really bad. He says to the nurse, "Just show us what Pop needs and we will do it." The nurses work with the family in demonstrating how to apply a soft brace and how to safely get José out of bed. Pain management strategies are discussed.

Families will have different preferences for information and for involvement in decision-making and may range from avoidance to active engagement. Benbassat, Pilpel, and Tidhar (1998) identified factors associated with preference for a passive role to include minority status, less education, elderly, and more severe illness. They concluded that desire for information was more universal but there was greater variability with preferred degrees of participation in decision-making.

Begin by assessing the level of involvement desired. Do they want in-depth information or just enough to understand? Do they want to be involved in collaborating on decisions related to treatment or delegate decision-making to health care providers? Recognize that these preferences are not constant but are likely to change as condition of the patient changes, families become more experienced with illness management, and other life circumstances intervene. An awareness of preferences will allow for tailoring of information as well as the level of decision-making.

Sobo (2004) emphasizes that preference for information may not be the same as preference for involvement in treatment decisions. Some families may engage in information exchange without decision-making whereas others may want to engage in both. In order to tailor the intervention to be appropriate to the patient and family, the nurse should ask the patient and/or family two clarifying questions about information and decision-making preferences.

1. When possible, what level of information would you prefer to receive?
   - The simplest information possible
   - More than the simplest information but keep it on everyday terms
   - In-depth information that you can help me understand
   - As much in-depth and detailed information as can be provided

2. When possible, what decision-making role do you (patient and/or family) want to assume?
   - Leave all decisions about care to the care team
   - Have the care team make decisions about care with serious consideration of our views
   - Share in making the decisions about care with the care team
   - Make all decisions about care with serious consideration of care team's advice
   - Make all decisions about care

With the answers to these two critical questions, the nurse can ask: Compared to what is desired, is the current level of information giving and decision-making on target?

Information Giving

A major family role is to advocate for the care required for their loved one. Information is critical to advocacy and decision-making yet the majority of the literature finds that families almost universally indicate that health care providers did not provide the needed information (Classen, 2000; Jeffers, 1998; Kawik, 1996; Sobo, 2004). Not only was the information not provided but studies show that there are incongruencies between what clinicians believe patients and/or families should know and what patients want to know. Families report that information presented is often confusing and unintelligible and insufficient to effectively engage the patient in health-care decisions (Pierce & Hicks, 2001). Effective information giving is correlated to greater satisfaction with care, less anxiety, and to greater adherence to therapeutic regimen (Edwards & Elwyn, 2001; Maly, Bourque, & Engelhardt, 1999).

Information giving is most effective when there is an established nurse-family relationship. Generally this relationship is formed informally and over time. However with shortened hospital stays and short medical visits, one cannot afford to wait for this relationship to form gradually. Nurses need to be approachable and proactive in their approach to forming patient and family relationships and in providing information. Families often do not know how to ask for what is needed or even what to ask for. Some families have had negative experiences when requesting information and hesitate to speak up, often take the path of least resistance, and don't articulate their needs. Recognize that it takes both energy and courage to speak up and request information or demand specific care interventions. Families fear alienating themselves from the very people that they rely on (Taylor, 2006).

Creating a culture that gives permission for families to disagree with or question the care received requires the nurses to adopt a family-centered approach. Respect for the family and interventions that are family inclusive are needed. In care planning, consider: How can I support the family today? What are they saying? What are they feeling? What are they not saying? As you interact with the family and have an opportunity to talk with them, focus in on what the experience must be like for the patient. Ask them: What is it like when . . . ? What do you find hardest? What are some of the most frustrating aspects of this hospitalization/this illness/this regimen? What would you like to see done differently? What information do you need to help you manage the situation? (Taylor, 2006). Support the family in their advocacy role after you have learned the family needs and concerns.

Incorporating the Family in Decision-Making

Family decision-making can be a highly stressful process. Do I have the information I need? How do I decide when there is no clear-cut answer? What if I make the wrong decision? These are common concerns, especially among families of acutely ill patients where high uncertainty and often risky decisions are made under conditions of high emotional stress and time constraints (Pierce & Hicks, 2001).

Traditionally, health care providers have held paternalistic attitudes, assuming that their professional expertise was enough rationale for imposing their views on a situation without consulting the patient or family. This paternalistic approach focused predominantly on the medical/scientific model of disease, that the health care provider knows best, and that the provider and patient/family share the same goals. This approach no longer is considered acceptable. A family-centered approach emphasizes the impact of the illness on the patient/family, the family's role in care provision and health promotion, and the values and preferences of both the patient and the family.

That patients and families are interested in nonpaternalistic approaches was confirmed by Schattner, Bronstein, and Jellin (2006) who examined what changes patients and their families wanted from health care; they found that increased information and autonomy were the most frequently cited desirable changes. Whitmer and colleagues (2005) also concluded that families want to be more involved with decision-making and that health care providers need to incorporate family interest into the decision-making process. Shared decision-making is the preferred mode of interaction.

Shared decision-making is a process based on mutual respect and partnership and the relationship between the health care provider and the patient/family is critical to success (Pierce & Hicks, 2001; Schattner et al., 2006). It requires patients and families to engage in conversation with nurses and physicians and make their view on well-being clear. Shared decision-making consists of discussions between professional and the patient/family that bring the knowledge, concerns, and perspective of each to the process of seeking agreement on a course of treatment. The focus of shared decision-making is to elicit the patient and family's perspective, understand the unique psychosocial context, reach a shared understanding concordant with patient and family values, and help patients and families to share power (de Haes, 2006).

Shared decision-making requires that a practitioner seek not only to understand each patient's needs and develop reasonable alternatives to meet those needs, but also to present the alternatives in a way that enables patients to choose one they prefer. Makoul and Clayman

(2006) identified the essential elements of shared decision-making to include:

- Definition/explanation of the problem
- Presentation of treatment options
- Discussion of pros and cons of treatment options on prognosis and quality of life
- Discussion of patient and family values/preferences
- Discussion of patient and family strengths, abilities, self-efficacy
- Discussion of nurse/physician recommendations
- Check and clarify patient and family understanding
- Make or explicitly defer the decision
- Arrange follow-up

In the three given case studies, the nursing staff successfully moved toward a family-centered paradigm with shared decision-making meeting the objectives of assisting the patients/families to obtain the information they need to participate at the level desired despite anxiety and uncertainty, reducing the psychological stress of making decisions, and helping patients/families arrive at decisions that accurately reflect their preferences and values. Each case presented unique challenges but the common theme was that the family did not expect a paternalistic approach but a team approach with the family assuming different levels of decision-making. Marie served as Lisa's surrogate during the coma period. She desired in-depth detailed information that she could discuss with the health care team and wanted to make decisions about care with serious consideration of the care team's advice. This very proactive role can be challenging for nurses and physicians more comfortable with the paternalistic approach. It led to strategies that likely had not yet been planned by the nursing staff—removing the Foley as a precautionary measure to avoiding urinary tract infection, positioning Lisa in a chair while still comatose, and beginning more in-depth physical therapy on a preventative basis. Bill and Nancy participated in shared decision-making with the nurse practitioner. Nancy in particular wanted in-depth information that was presented in an understandable way that helped her to understand Bill's symptoms and treatment. José's family needed another style of interaction. They wanted more than the simplest information but kept on everyday terms. They were comfortable with the decisions about care being made by the health care team as long as the team accepted their preferences of nondisclosure and family-centered rather than individualistic approach to decision-making.

As shown in the three case studies, there is no universalistic approach to family involvement and decision-making apart from being proactive in establishing a respectful and inclusive relationship with the family. The nurse must assess the pressing concerns and needs of both the patient and family and determine their desired level for information giving and decision-making. Negotiating approaches based on the patient and families' desires will result in greater satisfaction, more in-depth knowledge of the patient and family context, and improved short-term as well as long-term patient outcomes.

References

Benbassat, J., Pilpel, D., Tidhar, M. (1998). Patients' preferences for participation in clinical decision-making: A review of published surveys. *Behavioral Medicine*, 24(2), 81–88.

Bruera, E., Sweeney, C., Calder, K., Palmer, L., Benisch-Tolley, S. (2001). Patient preferences versus physician perceptions of treatment decisions in cancer care. *Journal of Clinical Oncology*, 19(11), 2883–2885.

Burchard, D. J. (2005). Family nursing: Challenges and opportunities: What will the challenges for family nursing be over the next few years? *Journal of Family Nursing*, 11(4), 332–335.

Classen, M. (2000). A handful of questions: Supporting parental decision-making. *Clinical Nurse Specialist*, 14(4), 189–195.

Cook, D. (2001). Patient autonomy versus paternalism. *Critical Care Medicine*, 20(2), N24–N25.

Corlett, J., & Twycross, A. (2006). Negotiation of parental roles within family-centered care: A review of the research. *Journal of Clinical Nursing*, 15, 1308–1316.

de Haes, H. (2006). Dilemmas in patient centeredness and shared decision-making: A case for vulnerability. *Patient Education and Counseling*, 62, 291–298.

Edwards, A., & Elwyn, G. (2001). Developing professional ability to involve patients in their care: Pull or push? *Quality Health Care*, 10, 129–130.

Espezel, H., & Canam, C. (2003). Parent-nurse interactions: Care of hospitalized children. *Journal of Advanced Nursing*, 44, 34–41.

Friedman, M. M. (1998). *Family nursing: Research, theory, and practice* (4th ed.). Stamford, CT: Appleton & Lange.

Gerteis, M., Edgman-Levitan, S., Daley, J., & Delbanco, T. L. (1993). *Through the patient's eyes*. San Francisco: Jossey-Bass.

Grey, M., Knafl, K., & McCorkle, R. (2006). A framework for the study of self- and family management of chronic conditions. *Nursing Outlook*, 54(5), 278–286.

Hack, T. F., Degner, L. F., Watson, P., & Sinha, L. S. (2005). Do patients benefit from participating in medical decision-making? Longitudinal follow-up of women with breast cancer. *Psycho-Oncology*, 15, 9–19.

Jeffers, B. R. (1998). The surrogate's experience during treatment decision-making. *MedSurg Nursing*, 7(6), 357–363.

Kawik, L. (1996). Nurses' and parents' perceptions of participation and partnership in caring for a hospitalized child. *British Journal of Nursing, 5,* 593–602.

Kickbusch, I. (1996, November). *Setting health objectives: The health promotion challenge.* Keynote presentation at Healthy People 2000 Consortium Meeting, New York.

Leske, J. S. (1991). Overview of family needs after critical illness: From assessment to intervention. *AACN Clinical Issues Critical Care Nursing, 2,* 220–226.

Leske, J. S. (2002). Interventions to decrease family anxiety. *Critical Care Nurse, 22*(6), 61–65.

Makoul, G., & Clayman, M. L. (2006). An integrative model of shared decision-making in medical encounters. *Patient Education and Counseling, 60,* 301–312.

Maly, R. C., Bourque, L. B., & Engelhardt, R. F. (1999). A randomized controlled trial of facilitating information giving to patients with chronic medical conditions: Effects on outcomes of care. *Journal of Family Practice, 48*(5), 356–363.

Mitchell, M. L., Courney, M., & Coyer, F. (2003). Understanding uncertainty and minimizing families' anxiety at the time of transfer from intensive care. *Nursing and Health Sciences, 5,* 207–217.

Pierce, P. F., & Hicks, F. D. (2001). Patient decision-making behavior. *Nursing Research, 50*(5), 267–274.

Salmond, S., & Spears, J. (2002). Psychosocial care of clients and their families. In A. Maher, S. Salmond, & T. Pellino (Eds.). *Orthopaedic nursing* (3rd ed.), (pp. 26–29). Philadelphia: Saunders.

Schattner, A., Bronstein, A., & Jellin, N. (2006). Information and shared decision-making are top patients' priorities. *BMC Health Services Research, 6,* 21.

Sobo, E. J. (2004). Pediatric nurses may misjudge parent communication preferences. *Journal of Nursing Care Quality, 19*(3), 253–262.

Taylor, B. (2006). Giving children and parents a voice—The parents' perspective. *Paediatric Nursing, 18*(9), 20–23.

Whitmer, M., Hughes, B., Hurst, S. M., & Young, T. B. (2005). Innovative solutions: Family conference progress note. *Dimensions of Critical Care Nursing, 24*(2), 83–88.

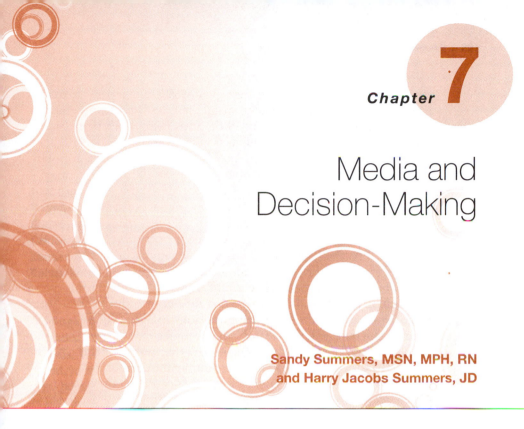

Sandy Summers, MSN, MPH, RN
and Harry Jacobs Summers, JD

Chapter 7

Media and Decision-Making

> **Four hostile newspapers are more to be feared
> than a thousand bayonets.**
>
> —Napoleon Bonaparte (1769–1821)

The modern media is pervasive and highly influential. It shapes our culture, our government, and our lives. English statesman Edmund Burke (1739–1797) termed the media the "fourth estate," when he proclaimed its strength greater than all the "three estates in Parliament" (Newspaper Association, 2005). Thousands of times every day, the media presents society with a persuasive vision of what society is, what it might be, and what it should be. The media investigates, hosts, and fosters public dialogue, and it regularly influences public decision-making, operating largely outside the domain of government officials in free societies.

The media does more than a government body. The media influences and even creates much of our culture. Its power lies in changing the way people think. U.S. advertisers spend $500 billion per year to buy media (Young, 2006). Those who spend these vast sums clearly believe that people will take actions based on advertising's persuasive, one-sided flows of information on subjects where viewers/readers may not have a great deal of prior experience or knowledge. This is also why powerful political ads can move polling numbers and affect election results. In addition, research shows that the news and entertainment media affect what people believe and how they act on a wide range of issues, including health-related issues.

Clearly, the media also has a tremendous impact on how the public sees health care, including nurses and nursing practice. At every moment of every day, the media sends the public powerful messages, not only about important issues like cancer or health insurance, but about who nurses are, what they know, what they do, and how much their work matters. These messages drive decision-making in all areas and at all levels, including the actions of patients, nurses and their colleagues, hospital managers, top federal officials and the voters who elect them. The media thus plays a critical role in shaping the current state of nursing care, and, particularly because the media's overall treatment of nursing is deeply flawed and damaging, it offers important avenues for nurses to improve their situation and the care of their patients.

This chapter starts with a case study that illustrates the media's effect on the population, the image of nurses in the media, and the work that nurses need to do to change that image so that they gain a respected place in health care decision-making. This chapter then presents a discussion about how nurses can use the media to increase their visibility, improve their image, and thus become valued decision-makers in health care.

Case Study

In November 2001, as part of the "Closing the Health Gap" campaign of the U.S. Department of Health and Human Services (HHS), the HHS Office of Minority Health (OMH) launched a new health initiative: the "Take a Loved One to the Doctor Day" campaign ("Loved One" campaign). The "Loved One" campaign was cofounded by HHS and ABC Radio's Urban Advantage Network, which has a weekly reach of more than 19 million listeners (HHS Press Office, 2004). The "Loved One" campaign's goal was to encourage members of minority populations to take charge of their personal health by educating and empowering them. The campaign would be held each year on the third Tuesday of September.

The "Loved One" campaign soon came to the attention of a small group of graduate students at the Johns Hopkins University School of Nursing. These students had just formed a group called the Nursing Vision. The purpose of the Nursing Vision was to increase public understanding of nursing and improve media images of nursing, which seemed especially urgent in view of the global nursing shortage. The group was concerned that the U.S. government would be promoting this worthy public health campaign with a name that excluded the work of the advanced practice registered nurses (APRNs) who provide a great deal of primary care to the underserved populations the campaign targets.

The "Loved One" issue came to the attention of the Nursing Vision and group members decided to take action. Several members sent letters and made telephone calls to the general number at OMH in early 2002, asking that the Office consider changing the campaign name to one that did not exclude APRNs.

When Sandy Summers, the Nursing Vision's cofounder, made a call to OMH, she was told that the office would never change the name of the campaign, because the word "doctor" tested so well in focus groups. After a time, the Nursing Vision set the matter aside, concluding that HHS was unlikely to change the name.

Later in 2002, Summers began to work full time on creating a more formal organization to address the widespread misunderstanding of nursing. The group incorporated, applied to the Internal Revenue Service for 501(c)(3) nonprofit status, and changed its name to the Center for Nursing Advocacy. Summers became the group's executive director. In late 2002, the Center launched a Web site, www.nursingadvocacy.org, on which it started analyzing nursing depictions in the media. The Center also began sending news alerts to supporters and encouraged them to send letters to the media to ask for more accurate depictions of nursing.

Soon, the Center began having some success in convincing corporations to end or modify advertising that used stereotypical images of nurses. A late 2003 *Washington Post* story covered the Center's campaign to convince the television show ER to depict nurses more accurately, and that story traveled across the globe (Center for Nursing Advocacy, 2003b). With experience and the increase in membership, the Center was becoming more effective.

In October 2004, the Center received a call from the American College of Nurse-Midwives (ACNM). ACNM remained concerned that the "Loved One" campaign name reinforced the damaging idea that only physicians provide primary care. The Center decided to renew its efforts to persuade OMH to change the name. The Center was now much larger, it had a powerful tool at its disposal—the web page from which a form e-mail letter could be sent. That tool had been essential to many of the Center's other successes.

Summers gathered information. She did research on the Internet and through calls to OMH collected the names and contact information of high-ranking individuals who would be involved in any decision to rename the campaign. This was a critical advocacy step—find the real decision-makers—and one that had not been employed in the Nursing Vision's 2002 efforts.

Summers also collected research comparing the care provided by physicians to the care provided by APRNs. The Center built a web page featuring the studies she found comparing the care of the two groups. The consensus of this research was that care provided by APRNs was as good as or better than that provided by physicians. This research would help to show why the "Loved One" campaign had no reason to exclude APRNs.

In the meantime, the ACNM drafted a proposed letter to OMH, which it sent to the Center for review in November 2004. In the letter, ACNM suggested five possible new names for the "Loved One" campaign, one of which was "Take a Loved One for a Checkup Day." The Center then drafted an analysis of the issue, which explained why the current name of the campaign was so damaging.

With the analysis ready, the Center prepared a letter to be sent to OMH. The Center embraced the ACNM's suggested name change of "Take a Loved One for a Checkup Day." On December 7, 2004, Summers e-mailed the letter to the Assistant Secretary for Minority Health and about seven other people at OMH, as well as the Secretary of HHS, and the host of a popular, nationally syndicated urban radio show, who had been the honorary chair of the "Loved One" campaign since its inception. Around this same time, ACNM and the American Academy of Nurse Practitioners (AANP) sent their own letters and urged their members to support the Center's campaign to have the name changed; a number of these members visited the Center's web site and sent letters using the site.

The Center also included a "Take Action" item on the "Loved One" campaign in its news alert of December 7. The item asked people to write to OMH and the other decision-makers. To make that easier, the item included a link to a proposed e-mail letter that had been adapted from the Center's letter to the decision-makers. Supporters were able to simply sign this form letter, or draft their own letter, then send the result to the decision-makers. On December 17, the Center issued a press release, but the media failed to pick up the story.

Letters from the Center's web site began rolling in to HHS from concerned nurses and supporters. The letters appeared to be reaching the e-mail inboxes of at least some of the decision-makers.

In mid-December 2004, Summers called OMH and asked to set up a telephone call with the Assistant Secretary for Minority Health, an executive who was relatively new to the job and had not been with

OMH in 2002. By this time, OMH had received about 200 letters from the Center's web site. After a number of requests, the call was arranged.

On December 21, Summers had a conference call with the Assistant Secretary and another OMH decision-maker. During the call, Summers explained the problem with the "Doctor Day" part of the campaign name and stressed how helpful a change would be. The Assistant Secretary was receptive, and he agreed to explore the idea of a name change. The Center kept the campaign open, and on January 3, 2005, Summers sent the Assistant Secretary an e-mail requesting more definitive action on OMH plans to change the "Doctor Day" name so the Center could end its campaign. Around this time, OMH staff members assured Summers that a letter from the Assistant Secretary would be forthcoming.

On January 12, 2005, American Nurses Association president Barbara Blakeney sent the HHS decision-makers a letter about the name change that was drawn largely from the center's model.

On January 28, 2005, the Assistant Secretary for Minority Health sent the Center and the other nursing groups a letter confirming that HHS working groups would seek a new name for the campaign. The Center ended its active campaign about the name. At this point, OMH had received about 370 letters from the Center's web site.

In July 2005, OMH began issuing materials relating to the upcoming September campaign day. These materials showed that OMH had changed the name to "Take a Loved One for a Checkup Day," as the Center and ACNM had suggested. The OMH campaign used that name in 2005 and 2006, and almost all of the campaign's media and health care partners used the new name as well. Unfortunately, the host of the popular syndicated show on ABC Radio's Urban Advantage Network, who continued to serve as honorary co-chair of the campaign, refused to use the new name. His office dismissed the Center's concerns, telling Summers in a phone call that the change could have "harmful effects" and that the original name had "capital." Thus, working for universal buy-in of the "Checkup Day" name continues to be an important goal for the Center going forward. (See **Figure 7-1**.)

This case study is an example of how one small group decided to take action and place constructive pressure on a very powerful second group. This pressure, applied via the use of media strategies, caused a shift in the second group's perceptions, resulting in a decision to change the name of a prominent national media campaign. The tactics used may be applied in any venue where the message of the media would help effect positive change. The change in the title of this media campaign gave the public greater awareness of and thus access to health care providers other than the "doctor," and it potentially improved understanding of the value of nurses and their ability to be included as decision-makers in health care.

Figure 7-1

A "Loved One" campagin ad, with name changed.

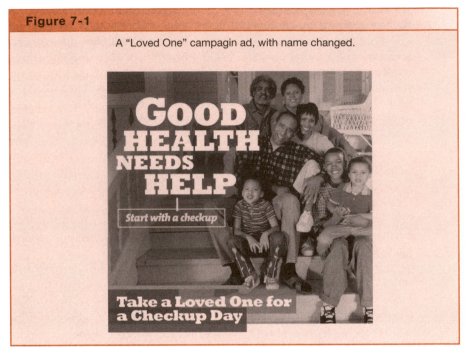

Source: U.S. Department of Health and Human Services.

The Pervasive Influence of the Media

The average American spends 3,518 hours per year, or 60 percent of that person's awake time, consuming media (U.S. Census Bureau, 2007). Research shows that this media—including advertising and entertainment programming—has a significant impact on what consumers think and do. Nurses therefore have an enormous opportunity to bring messages about nursing and health care generally to patients and society at large by tapping into the insatiable desire for media entertainment and information. Unfortunately, although there have been accurate and helpful depictions of nursing, too much of the media's depiction of the profession has been damaging. This poor depiction affects the public's ideas about the value of nursing, and about nurses' role and influence in health care decision-making.

Effects of Media on Health Care and Nursing

In recent years, a consensus has emerged in the field of public health, based on considerable research, that what people see in the media has a significant effect on their health-related views and behavior. A wide range of public agencies, private groups, and scholars now devote substantial resources to analyzing and managing health messages in the media. This is part of the public health field called *health communications*.

Health communications is a "hybrid" with roots in communications, health care, and other fields (Glik, 2003). Glik (2003) states that health communications contain both planned and unplanned messages that can be positive, neutral, or negative. These unplanned messages are significant in that people are influenced by media content whether or not the creators specifically intended that they take away the message received.

What the media tells people about health care works much like advertising. As one public health scholar noted "[f]rom a social marketing perspective, messages in the media that promote specific desirable behaviors have the potential to persuade consumers to change their behavior if messages are viewed as compatible with consumers' own self-interest, competing messages are minimal, and resistance to change is low to moderate" (Glik, 2003, p. 1).

News media coverage also affects the public's perception and beliefs about health care (Turow & Gans, 2002). Because treatment of health topics in the news media has a significant effect on public views and actions, advocates have worked hard to affect the frequency and accuracy of the media's coverage of health topics in which they have an interest (Glik, 2003).

Media influence is hardly confined to hard-news outlets. On the contrary, what people see in the fictional media has a significant effect on their health-related views and behavior as well. In 2000, the U.S. Centers for Disease Control and Prevention surveyed prime-time TV viewers and found that most (52%) reported getting information that they trust to be accurate from prime-time TV shows (Henry J. Kaiser Family Foundation, 2004). More than a quarter of this survey's respondents said such shows were among their top three sources for health information (Henry J. Kaiser, 2004). Nine out of 10 regular viewers said they learned something about diseases or disease prevention from television, with almost half citing prime-time or daytime entertainment shows (Henry J. Kaiser, 2004). Moreover, almost half of regular viewers who heard something about a health issue on a prime-time show said they took one or more actions, including telling someone about the storyline (42%), telling someone to do something (such as using a condom or getting more exercise) or doing it themselves (16%), or visiting a clinic (9%) (Henry J. Kaiser, 2004).

Some research has focused on the effects of specific shows, particularly the popular NBC drama ER. This show has been on the air since 1994 and is now shown in many nations around the world. During the U.S. television seasons running during 1997–2000, the Henry J. Kaiser Family Foundation surveyed 3,500 regular ER viewers (Brodie et al., 2001; Henry J. Kaiser, 2003; Henry J. Kaiser, 2002). In the Kaiser surveys, more than half (53%) of regular ER viewers said they learned about important health issues while watching the show. Almost a third said information from the show helped them make choices about their own family's health care; this was especially true of viewers with less-formal education (44% with no college versus 25% with some college). As a result of watching ER, almost a quarter of viewers said they sought further information about a health issue, and 14 percent actually contacted a health care provider because of something they saw in an ER episode.

At least one study suggested a link between public attitudes toward nursing and ER. In a 2000 JWT Communications focus group study of youngsters in grades 2–10, respondents said they received their main impression of nursing from ER (JWT Communications, 2000). Consistent with the show's physician-centric approach, the young people also wrongly believed that nursing was a girl's job, that it was a technical job "like shop," and that it was an inappropriate career for private school students, of whom more was expected (JWT Communications, 2000).

Nursing's Role in Shaping Health Messages

Nurses can help to shape health messages for public consumption. However, the profession's public image may actually impede nurses' efforts to play this role.

Although nurses commonly top polls measuring which professions are the most trusted, any serious evaluation of the profession's public image reveals that most people do not understand what nurses actually do or why nursing work matters (Center for Nursing Advocacy, 2006a). On the contrary, nursing's public image has long been based primarily on stereotypes, including the physician's handmaiden, the angel, and the "naughty nurse" (Center, 2007b; Center, 2007c; Darbyshire & Gordon, 2005; Kalisch & Kalisch, 1986). Thus, while nurses have tended to enjoy public affection, they have not received the real respect that might lead to a better allocation of clinical, educational, and research resources for the profession or allow nurses a real seat at the table of policy-making and clinical decision-making. Nurses' image as workers without significant knowledge also has negatively impacted the public's perception of the validity of information that nurses offer them for health decision-making, both on an individual basis and in wider public forums. To take just one example, consider the primitive depictions of family presence on television dramas, which regularly feature physicians ordering family members far away from patient bedsides during emergency procedures as a matter of course, as if no one had ever questioned this practice. If nurses had meaningful input, it seems likely that such influential shows would be giving the public a better sense of evolving health practices in this regard (Center, 2006g).

Since research shows that the media has such a strong influence on public understanding of nursing and health care in general, it is vital to nursing and public health that nurses improve their media image. Indeed, if the mass media is critical to modern health strategies overall, then it must also be a key means of addressing one of the most important worldwide health problems: the nursing shortage.

Media Portrayal of Nurses: The Stereotypes

The media frequently portrays nursing work because nursing involves life, death, conflict and drama—the stuff of compelling and important media. Unfortunately, the media commonly portrays nurses stereotypically, often crediting physicians for their work, and this is especially true of the most influential media, television. Factors contributing to this may include entrenched social biases (including gender bias) and assumptions about nursing, including:

- The view that smart, ambitious women with an interest in health care necessarily become physicians
- What one scholar has called nursism, a more general social bias against the caring role that contributes negatively to the way nursing is perceived (Lewenson, 1993)
- The media's common reliance on well-understood (but often incorrect) conventions
- A lack of significant support for nursing from the physicians who continue to exercise great influence over the media and who enjoy unparalleled esteem, including the widespread assumption that they provide all important health care
- Nursing's own failure to adequately represent itself to the media and the public at large (Buresh & Gordon, 2006)

There have been notable exceptions, particularly in the print media, in documentaries, and a few fictional products (Center, 2006b). However, the overall impression of nursing the public gets from the media is distorted and inadequate to the needs of nurses and their patients.

The most common nursing stereotypes are:

- **The Physician Handmaiden.** Nurses have long been portrayed as fungible females who have no great level of training, no unique scope of practice, and no significant role in substantive health care. Instead, they are seen to exist to help the physicians who do provide important health care; it is assumed that physicians supervise and manage nurses and know everything nurses do. This is perhaps the most damaging stereotype, because it remains so common and so persuasive to a public that knows little of what nurses really do. Indeed, the handmaiden remains the central nursing image in popular Hollywood television shows, where the few nurses who appear seem to exist to get physicians or get things for physicians. Handmaiden images range from the less-obviously damaging portrayals of nurses as skilled physician subordinates, as seen on shows like ER and Scrubs, to the explicit attacks on the profession in products like Grey's Anatomy or House, where nurses tend to be clueless, often disagreeable servants who represent everything ambitious modern women have left behind (Center, 2006c).

The "Naughty Nurse." The "naughty nurse" image commonly takes the form of a female model or actress dressed in a supposed "nursing uniform" that amounts to lingerie. Such images remain a staple of media communications of the advertising, apparel, hospitality, and entertainment industries, particularly in products directed at younger males. Some entertainment programming continues to suggest that nurses tend to be sexually available to physicians, one example being the depiction of "skanky syph[ilis] nurse" Olivia on Grey's Anatomy. The Center for Nursing Advocacy (discussed in the earlier case study) has convinced many corporate advertisers to reconsider such images, though the images continue to appear in prominent media worldwide. As the Center explained, even though these images are often "jokes" or "fantasies," the stereotypes they promote discourage practicing and potential nurses, encourage sexual violence in the workplace, and contribute to a general atmosphere of disrespect that make it difficult for nurses to get the respect and resources they need (Center, 2006d).

The Angel. On the surface, the image of nurses as angels is seemingly the best of the stereotypes, and some nurses themselves endorse it. Indeed, the angel image is fueled by some media products that are designed to appeal to nurses, such as uniforms. However, the image of nurses as devoted handholders and scut-work saints undervalues nurses' knowledge and advanced skills. It may also allow decision-makers to discount poor working conditions that nurses endure or to treat the conditions as evidence of nurses' virtue, rather than problems that must be addressed. Some nurses, including the Center for Nursing Advocacy, view the Johnson & Johnson (J&J) Campaign for Nursing's Future television commercials as employing this stereotype. These nurses note that a trusted, baby-soft image is obviously helpful to a major pharmaceutical corporation, which benefits by aligning itself with a profession at the pinnacle of public trust, but that nursing itself is not well-served by the perpetuation of the view that nurses are relatively unskilled spiritual beings with no earthly needs (Center, 2006I).

The Battleaxe. The "battleaxe" image essentially presents the nurse as an unattractive, bitter, and malevolent force, often the representation of an unfeeling bureaucracy or institutional oppression. This image continues to appear from time to time in advertising and entertainment programming. The image may stem in part from a need to compensate for a feeling that female nurses may have significant power over vulnerable men in clinical settings, and from a belief that any assertive nurse who fails to conform to the more submissive nursing stereotypes must be a she-demon. Nurse Ratched from *One Flew Over the Cuckoo's Nest* is perhaps the best-known example of the battleaxe, a portrayal that may be the most influential modern image of a nurse who seems to delight in torturing patients. The book and film are assigned to college students across the land, and these artistic and culturally significant works are likely to help perpetuate the battleaxe image for decades to come (Center for Nursing Advocacy, 2003a).

The Physician Golddigger or "Wannabe Mrs. Kovac." This image has long existed in tandem with the strand of the "naughty nurse" image that presents the nurse as being sexually available to physicians. Recent examples include remarks by television psychologist "Dr. Phil" McGraw in 2004, who suggested on the air that the health care system is full of "cute little nurses" who are out to "seduce and marry" physicians "because that's their ticket out of having to work as a nurse." Dr. Phil later made on-air statements expressing support for nursing after the center contacted the show and the show received more than 1,400 letters sent through the Center's Web site (Center for Nursing Advocacy, 2004b).

The Female Caregiver. Even a casual look at the preceding images shows that the most common nursing stereotypes are closely linked to the prevailing assumption that nurses are female caregivers. In the JWT Communications (2000) research of 1,800 U.S. school children in grades 2–10, researchers found that when the focus groups' topic changed to nursing, the boys stopped paying attention, as if the conversation no longer pertained to them. It has been persuasively argued that caregiving has long been admired, but rarely considered intellectually challenging or truly essential outside of the family structure (Nelson & Gordon, 2006). Although there has been recent media about men in nursing and a few minor nurse characters in recent Hollywood shows have been male, major depictions of nurses remain overwhelmingly female. Of course, nursing does remain less than 10 percent male (U.S. Department of Health and Human Services, 2000). However, as long as it is portrayed as a profession that is for "caring" females, it will be considered work that is too effeminate and insubstantial for men—and too lowly for anyone interested in an autonomous, challenging career.

Any Helpful Person or Thing Is a Nurse. The media, notably in promoting recent feature films like The Skeleton Key (2005), has tended to suggest that nursing is something any caring person can do—that any caregiver is a "nurse." Consider the recent growth in "baby nurses," who are actually nannies for newborns who may have no health care training at all. Still, these workers commonly refer to themselves—and are referred to in the major media—by the shorthand "nurse." After one "baby nurse" allegedly injured a newborn in New York in 2005, the state legislature passed a law to prevent nonnurses from calling themselves "nurses" (Center, 2005a). In 2006, the CVS pharmaceutical chain featured a television commercial in which a pharmacist suggested that by helping a patient's spouse learn about her complex medication regimen in half a day, he had turned the spouse into a nurse. After a few calls from the center, CVS removed this statement from its commercial (Center, 2006h). Another common version of this image appears when makers of electronic health care tools that perform relatively simple tasks market their products with names like "electronic nurse," or otherwise suggest that the product will be acting as a nurse, as has been the case with some surgical robots. The media is often eager to call such machines "nurses" (Center, 2006l). The Center has convinced a number of these creators to cease naming their products after skilled nurses.

The Wallpaper Nurse. Nurse characters populate the background of popular television shows like House doing busy work as a kind of garnish to the glamorous, important work of the heroic physicians on which the camera focuses. These "wallpaper nurses" may morph out of the background to push gurneys, deliver messages, or hand things to physicians. They often are presented as mute automatons who would seem not to need significant education or resources; certainly few viewers would want to see themselves in such a role. Ironically, the actors playing these roles are often real nurses.

The Physician Nurse. Physician characters on fictional television shows are often presented performing the work that real-life nurses do. There are about 30 major characters on the four top U.S. hospital shows (*Grey's Anatomy*, *House*, *ER*, and *Scrubs*). All but two of these characters are physicians. Because the majority of real hospital work is done by nurses, including tasks involving patient interactions and many of the key tasks in critical procedures, the media's physician characters must do nursing jobs just to make the shows' drama work. This effectively gives physicians credit for the exciting work that nurses really do. At the same time, the news media commonly consults only physicians for advice in areas where nurses generally have greater expertise, such as breastfeeding, pain management, and patient education.

The Cut-Rate Physician Substitute. A large body of research shows that the care of APRNs is *at least* as good as that provided by physicians (Center, 2006e), yet media entities often present items that ignore the very existence of APRNs, even in areas where APRNs play a central role, such as primary care for underserved populations. In 2005, the Center and other nurses persuaded the U.S. Department of Health and Human Services to change the name of its annual minority health campaign from "Take a Loved One to the Doctor Day" to "Take a Loved One for a Checkup Day," as noted in the case study (Center, 2005b). The news media may also accept criticism of APRN care by competitors in organized medicine with little or no question, as has often occurred in connection with the growth of APRN-staffed retail-based clinics. Such press pieces often do not even consult APRNs (Center, 2006k).

The prevalence of these stereotypes has a significant negative impact on health care decision-making and nursing. When nurses are seen mainly as low-skilled physician subordinates, their health care expertise has less impact on colleagues, patients, the media, and the public. Nurses also struggle to get the resources they need to provide high-quality direct care, to conduct vital research, and to educate a new generation of nurses.

The Challenge of Getting "Real Nursing" into the Media

The question remains: How do we get real nursing into the media, so we can change the population's perception of nursing? This is essential if the voice of nursing in the shaping of health care is to be heard, or at the very least, so the population served values nurses' information and applies it in day-to-day health decision-making. To improve public understanding of nursing and improve health care itself, nurses must become more involved in shaping the media that the public consumes—yet getting nursing into the media is a monumental challenge. Nurses have been reluctant to step forward and reach out to the media. At the same time, the media has failed to seek out nurses for their expert comment, instead consulting physicians on subjects for which nurses are generally more expert. This is presumably a result of the cumulative effect of the stereotypical nursing image just discussed, but it may stem in particular from the belief that nursing is merely a minor subset of medicine, rather than a separate, autonomous profession (Center, 2006f). When nurses have so little independent credibility in the media, it is hard for them to be seen as reliable, knowledgeable health resources by and for their patients.

The Process of Communicating

In mass communication, there is typically a sender, a message, a recipient, and feedback (Reynolds, 1997). The message is crafted to reach certain types of recipients; often, it is aimed at a specific demographic. The message is sent in a specific medium, with the sender making an effort to cut through background noise and clutter. Recipients decode the message in their own way based on the message, the clutter, and the level of credibility of the sender, which affects whether recipients take action on the message in accord with the sender's goals (Freed, 2006).

Under this framework, nurses who wish to communicate must assess their credibility as health educators. Of course, Gallup polls show nurses have a high level of public trust (Saad, 2006)—but trust is not the same as respect. Based on the rampant negative media depictions and relatively low funding for the profession as a whole, it seems that the public trusts nurses to hold their wallets while they are in surgery, but not to play a significant role in keeping patients alive while they are actually in surgery or to educate them about how to recover. True respect for the profession would entail meaningful public inquiry into the nature of nursing work and the people who do it. It would mean serious federal funding to address the global nursing shortage—one of the greatest public health crises in today's world. It would mean incorporation of nurses on every board and committee related to health. It would mean that at least half of every hospital board was composed of nurses. However, because nursing is undervalued, these things are not happening.

The bedrock components of nursing practice are direct patient care, patient education, and patient advocacy. Nursing education, nursing research, and nursing advocacy underpin each of the three components. When nurses advocate for a stronger profession, they are improving their direct care and their ability to educate and advocate for patients. If nurses wish to increase the number of people who take positive action based on their health messages, they must increase their credibility as health educators—and that begins with improving their media image.

If nurses continue to avoid participating in the media, they will miss vital opportunities to reach patients and society with key health information, including information to help the public better understand nursing itself. Patients will lack the information they need to make good health decisions. In recent years, some nurses have worked effectively to communicate about their work, through media such as books, radio shows, op-ed pieces, and public advocacy campaigns (Center, 2006b; 2007a). However, the profession must be far more vocal and assertive if it is to make the sea change in public understanding that the current situation requires.

Nurses Must Improve Nursing's Image in Order to Improve Health Care

Some might ask why nurses have to improve the nursing image in order to get key health messages to patients and the public. The reason is that when nursing is so undervalued in the public consciousness—when people think that only physicians have substantive knowledge about health issues—then nurses' health messages are not heard or acted upon by patients.

Consider the last time you were at a family gathering, neighborhood cookout, or party. It is common for nurses to meet new people or old friends and have the conversation turn to personal health issues. In such situations, nurses have a great opportunity to educate people, one by one, about health issues, and also to establish themselves as health experts. Family, friends, or acquaintances might tell a nurse of their health concerns, and particularly given nursing's strong focus on preventative health and health management, the nurse might be eager to educate as well as possible given the social setting. However, many nurses report that social bias or nursism can work against them in these settings. Nurses often have the sense that their messages are not heard, believed or adopted, even though they were based on evidence and years of advanced training, particularly if the nursing advice appears to be inconsistent with that of a physician.

It would hardly take a logical leap to surmise that the basic reason for this lack of perceived credibility is the huge gulf in the levels of genuine social respect for medicine and nursing. Because nurses are constantly seen as people who do not know anything meaningful or substantive, their expert advice is often ignored or discounted—and needless to say, this problem exists in clinical settings as well; nurses often have the sense that what they tell patients and non-nurse colleagues is discounted in critical decision-making. However, neither patients nor colleagues can afford to undervalue nurses' teaching. It is vital to public health that these recipients hear and heed nurses' messages, many of which the recipients are unlikely to hear anywhere else—and many of which could make the difference between life and death.

If nurses want to reach out to the media and start affecting it, they need to know the nuts and bolts of how the media works. What follows are suggestions to do just this, using the media as a way to educate the populations that nurses serve in their own everyday decision-making.

Every nurse should read and consider the advice in *From Silence to Voice* by Bernice Buresh and Suzanne Gordon, now in its second edition (2006). The authors, experienced journalists who serve on the Center's board of directors, have written a fabulous how-to manual on how the media works and how nurses can better participate in media coverage. This important book shows that nurses have not given the public an adequate account of their work, but it offers strategies to help nurses tell the world what they do, in order to get the resources and respect needed to resolve the nursing crisis and help patients achieve better health.

Interested nurses should also read the excellent fifth edition (2007) of *Policy & Politics in Nursing and Health Care*, edited by Diana Mason, Judith Leavitt, and Mary Chaffee. Especially helpful is Chapter 9: "Harnessing the Power of the Media to Influence Health Policy and Politics" that features information on getting free media coverage, Internet activism, "Talking the Right Talk" by Suzanne Gordon, and a segment on the work of the Center (Mason, Dodd, & Glickstein, 2007).

Nurses who believe they may have the opportunity to speak to the media should consider getting media training. Nurses' employers can encourage such training, and perhaps pay for the costs, in order to help nurses increase understanding of their work and promote the institution by extension. In fact, institutions might consider maintaining a core group of nurses who are skilled at interacting with the media. The Center's media-training resources page, www.nursingadvocacy.org/action/media_training.html, has links to discussions of media myths, media training seminars and workshops, and online resources. Nurses can also get tips on writing powerful letters in the Center's guide at www.nursingadvocacy.org/action/get_help_writing.html.

The following are some specific strategies nurses might use to persuade society that they and their messages are worthy of attention.

Reaching Out to the Media

To get media coverage, nurses must actively seek it. As Buresh and Gordon (2006) show, nurses have traditionally shied away from the media in accord with the prevailing "virtue script," which entails a code of self-effacement. Naturally, physicians and others have been happy to supply the media with input that nurses have declined to provide. This system has not served the profession of nursing well, so nurses must work to make sure they are seen and heard.

Appoint a Public Relations Professional to Promote Nursing

One way to get the word out about the work that nurses do at an institution is to appoint a public relations (PR) person who is dedicated *solely* to that task. Many hospitals have one or more PR professionals who promote physicians and the hospital in general, but there is rarely a focus on nursing. However, Massachusetts General Hospital (MGH) has a PR person dedicated to promoting *only* nursing at the hospital. Other hospitals should be encouraged to follow this example. In October 2005, the *Boston Globe* published an excellent four-part, front-page series on the training of a new ICU nurse. In order to get the story, the *Globe* reporter and photographer spent 9 months following a veteran nurse and her apprentice at MGH. That article was the result of significant effort by MGH's PR director for nursing Georgia Peirce, a member of the Center's board of directors, who spent months convincing the *Globe* to follow nurses and report on their work.

Provide News Resources for the Media

Individual nurses should offer to serve as expert resources for the media. In doing so, nurses should take care to be responsive, reliable, and credible. Specific measures nurses might consider to do this more effectively include:

- Collecting and promoting story ideas to help the media develop stories on nursing, and incorporate a nursing perspective in general health care stories

- Building a database of information on local nursing issues to use as a resource for responding to media inquiries
- Creating a roster of nurses who are expert in different fields to have on hand when the media does ask for expert input
- Developing online video news programs or Internet Web sites that depict real images of nursing
- Determining who a media entity's gate keeper or decision-maker is, and arranging to speak to that person
- Issuing press releases that create a framework for a story about nursing and health

One impressive example of this kind of media outreach is the work of the *American Journal of Nursing (AJN)* under the leadership of editor-in-chief Diana J. Mason, who sits on the Center's advisory panel. *AJN* has done a fabulous job of communicating with the general media about nursing research and other material appearing in the journal. The *AJN* creates press releases about significant material it runs and regularly contacts the media to pitch stories of interest. A compelling narrative story from *AJN* was republished in the November 2004 *Reader's Digest*, with readership around 80 million (Answers, 2007; Center for Nursing Advocacy, 2004a). The story told how one nurse spurred a declining leukemia patient's recovery after a bone marrow transplant by subtly getting him to engage with her over a cup of tea. The type of media outreach *AJN* does is the method used by physician journals, which is one reason their research receives such widespread press coverage.

Creating Media with Accurate Depictions of Nurses

Nurses must develop media that gives the public an accurate vision of the profession, including both its achievements and its problems. Many types of media can reach out to patients and educate them about health topics or nursing. For example, advertising can be very effective, especially when there is a good match between the medium, the message, and the resources of the advertiser. Television is a powerful way to communicate basic ideas, but it can be expensive unless a broadcaster donates the airtime. It appears to be easier to get donated radio airtime as compared to television. In 2005, the Ad Council reported $1 billion worth of donated radio time, $338 million worth of television and cable airtime, and $30 million worth of space donated by newspapers (Ad Council, 2006). Major newspapers and other publications can reach a significant audience with more complex messages, but they can be expensive. Radio and the Internet may be more affordable ways to reach certain audiences.

Society needs to know that nurses are experts in clinical practice and in health education. Potential ways to advance those goals include health education videos, articles, books (fiction and nonfiction), short stories, guides, television shows, movies (features, shorts, documentaries, animated), novels, plays, poems, Web sites, radio programs, paintings, comics, cartoons, children's interactive CDs (like *Rescue Heroes* for nurses), children's books, children's videos, coloring books, Halloween costumes, dolls, action figures, toys, and board games. Although such media might help to interest career seekers, the profession also needs nurses to create media that presents the challenges and problems that nursing confronts today. See more on creating nursing media at www.nursingadvocacy.org/create/create.html.

An example of a paid advertising campaign with major television and Internet components is Johnson & Johnson's prominent Campaign for Nursing's Future, whose stated goal has been to increase interest in nursing careers. Some elements of this campaign, particularly elements of the campaign's web site (partly created by the Center) and a short video about nurse scientists, contain helpful and persuasive information. As discussed earlier, some believe that the campaign's more influential television advertising spots tend to reinforce angel and handmaiden imagery but J&J has cited research suggesting that its campaign has significantly raised the profile of nursing in certain segments of the community (Center, 2006j).

Of course, shaping the course of existing media activity (paid and unpaid) remains critical because of that media's vast influence, and the fact that it constantly portrays health care, including nurses and nursing. The work of nursing so often is the subject of media attention because it is dramatic and exciting, filled with both intense emotion and cutting-edge technology, life and death, hope and despair. Influencing this media is often the most effective and affordable way to affect the nursing image and to deliver key health messages. Moreover, one of the best ways to advance any cause is earned media; press that those with a given interest generate by doing newsworthy things and encouraging the press to cover them. Of course, media created by those who are not seen to share a specific policy agenda (such as advancing nursing or some health message) can have more credibility with the public. Nurses can make claims about their work, but what the public sees about nursing in major newspapers (or Hollywood dramas) may be taken as a more objective account of the profession.

Though shaping existing media activity does not require direct payments, it can require a tremendous expenditure of time, effort, and skill, as evidenced by the case study presented at the beginning of the chapter. It can take years and more to make a change. The media rarely approaches nurses and asks them how it should portray them or health care generally. Therefore, nurses must work for better treatment of the health issues that matter to them.

Present a Professional Image of Nursing

Before nurses can expect to improve nursing's image, they must examine the image that each of them presents to the world. Some nurses may think professionalism means conforming to a traditional ideal of appearance, such as the white-starched apron and cap. Others may adopt a strict approach toward colleagues, patients, and families, imposing needless restrictions to maintain order, yet many professionals would not define their professions in these terms, but in terms of an unflagging commitment to the best interests of those they serve.

Part of any profession's image relates to the appearance of its members, and this may be particularly true for groups that do not enjoy automatic respect. If nurses want respect, they should strive to look like college-educated science professionals, as physicians and others in the clinical setting do. Some nurses wear patterned scrubs, and of course, the media often portrays nurses as doing so. One late 2006 episode of ER presented a resident physician who was mortified that, because her usual clothes had become messy at the hospital, she had to wear patterned scrubs that made her look like a nurse. Unsurprisingly, she was mocked by another physician. Many feel that patterned scrubs say "disrespect me!" to the public, just as the similar-looking 1960s housedresses said about homemakers.

Another important element of nurses' professional appearance is recognition in clinical settings that a nurse actually is a nurse. This is especially important because of the recent proliferation of other hospital workers, particularly unlicensed assistive personnel who may do tasks formerly done by nurses. Nurses need to take ownership of their own image, and it is not in the profession's interest for nurses to be confused with others in the clinical setting. Nurses should consider wearing the "RN" patch created in 2003 by Mark Dion and J. Morgan Puett, in collaboration with the Fabric Workshop and Museum in Philadelphia. The Center has crafted various versions of the RN patch for nurses with different educational credentials to help teach patients (and remind fellow health professionals) that it takes rigorous education to become a nurse. See more on uniforms and the RN patches at www.nursingadvocacy.org/action/RN_patch.html.

Nurses and others should also consider what messages their choice of language may send. When we suggest "nurse-friendly" language, we of course do not mean language that is nice to nurses, but language that reflects recognition that nurses are highly skilled health professionals who save lives and improve outcomes. (Similarly, "user-friendly" does not mean language that is nice to users, but language that helps them work effectively.) The nurse-friendly language section on frequently asked questions on the Center's Web site encourages the use of language that sends an accurate message about nurses and their role in health care. Some questions tackled are: "Are nurses who don't work at the bedside 'real nurses'?" "Should we refer to physician or nurse practitioner care plans as 'orders' (or prescriptions)?" See more on nurse-friendly language at www.nursingadvocacy.org/faq/nf/nf.html.

Nursing's Influence on the Health Care Decisions of Others

If nurses succeed in reducing the impact of the current stereotypes of their profession, nurses' voices will increasingly be recognized for what they are, and not seen as the natterings of some degraded fictional vision of nursing. Nurses then will be seen as valuable and reliable sources of information who can guide others in making important health decisions.

However, nurses must keep in mind that engaging with health-related media entails both opportunities and responsibilities. If the lay media is currently covering a health story or piece of research, people are very likely to start asking health professionals about it. At least 80 percent of adults who use the Internet have done so to research health issues, and health care information is the third most common reason for these adults' Internet usage (Pew Internet & American Life Project, 2003). Few nurses have been spared probing questions from Internet-educated patients about diseases or other health topics. Nurses must make efforts to stay connected to the information that the individuals they serve are accessing, so that nurses are conversant with new developments and able to respond to questions and concerns. Of course, it can be dangerous to rely on a lay media reporter's interpretation of a health care study, so nurses should go straight to the research when getting health information to make sure they understand and can explain it to patients better. Lay media articles almost always include the name of the underlying resource—usually a published article in a health care journal. Most hospitals and schools have subscriptions to major databases so nurses can access articles at no cost. Connecting patients to evidence-based information is critical to nurses' role in helping them make health care decisions.

Not all health-related media on the Internet is as accurate as it should be. When people come to nurses with health information from the Internet, nurses might advise them to look for the logo of the Health on the Net Foundation, an international nonprofit organization that works to verify the reliability of Internet health information. Information on the organization can be found at www.hon.ch. Readers can look for the Health on the Net logo, and click on it at a given web site to verify that the site is registered with the organization. If so, readers can have some confidence that the web site at least strives to deliver accurate and evidence-based health care information.

Nurses also must take active steps to shape the health information individuals see on the Internet and in other media. If the information is not accurate or complete, nurses should try to provide better information by working with the media using the suggestions given previously.

Send Feedback to the Media

It is important that nurses let the media know that they are watching, and that they expect the media to present a fair and accurate account of the profession, especially at a time when nursing is under great stress. Nurses should monitor the media and send feedback. Some examples include sending thanks to the media for accurate or three-dimensional coverage of nursing issues; providing feedback to journalists, individuals, or groups who are responsible for inaccurate or damaging depictions of nurses, as the case study presented earlier illustrates; and mobilize colleagues to protest poor portrayals of nursing.

Remember that even the entertainment and advertising media have powerful effects on public views of nursing and health, and many people are more likely to engage with health issues that are set in the context of popular entertainment. Many of us are more focused on what's happening on *Grey's Anatomy* than we are on the nightly news, and calling attention to how such entertainment products treat nursing can generate vital public discussion of nursing and its situation.

Conclusion

The media influences health care decisions, so nurses have an important responsibility to advocate for more accurate media depictions of nurses and nursing, as well as more accurate and complete messages that will support better decision-making in health care generally. As the "Take a Loved One for a Checkup Day" campaign shows, changing social perceptions through the media takes time, commitment, and a sustained, cohesive strategy. However, nurses *can* do it.

References

Ad Council. (2006). *PSA bulletin: 2005 record-breaking year in donated media*. Retrieved February 14, 2007, from www.adcouncil.org/psab/2006_July_August
Answers. (2007.) *Reader's Digest*. Retrieved February 15, 2007, from www.answers.com/topic/reader-s-digest

Brodie, M., Foehr, U., Rideout, V., Baer, N., Miller, C., Flournoy, R., & Altman, D. (2001). Communicating health information through the entertainment media. *Health Affairs, 20*(1), 192–199. Retrieved February 19, 2007, from http://content.healthaffairs.org/cgi/reprint/20/1/192

Buresh, B., & Gordon, S. (2006). *From silence to voice: What nurses know and must communicate to the public,* 2nd ed. Ithaca, NY: ILR Press.

Center for Nursing Advocacy. (2003a). *One flew over the cuckoo's nest review.* Retrieved February 19, 2007, from www.nursingadvocacy.org/media/films/cuckoos_nest.html

Center for Nursing Advocacy. (2003b). *Washington Post highlights center's "ER" campaign.* Retrieved February 25, 2007, from www.nursingadvocacy.org/news/2003nov18_washpost.html

Center for Nursing Advocacy. (2004a). *Killers, tea and sympathy.* Retrieved February 15, 2007, from www.nursingadvocacy.org/news/2004nov/rd.html

Center for Nursing Advocacy. (2004b). *Kicking Dr. Phil's ass to the curb.* Retrieved February 19, 2007, from www.nursingadvocacy.org/news/2004nov/18_dr_phil.html

Center for Nursing Advocacy. (2005a). *Take a loved one for a checkup day.* Retrieved February 11, 2007, from www.nursingadvocacy.org/news/2005jul/loved_one.html

Center for Nursing Advocacy. (2005b). *Babynewspaper.* Retrieved February 19, 2007, from www.nursingadvocacy.org/news/2005dec/04_balt_sun.html

Center for Nursing Advocacy. (2006a). *Why aren't you more excited that public opinion polls often put nurses at the top of the list of "most trusted" and "most ethical" professions?* Retrieved February 14, 2007, from www.nursingadvocacy.org/faq/most_trusted.html

Center for Nursing Advocacy. (2006b). *Golden lamp awards: Best media depictions of nursing 2006."* Retrieved February 14, 2007, from www.nursingadvocacy.org/press/releases/golden/2006/awd.html#best

Center for Nursing Advocacy. (2006c). *ER television review.* Retrieved February 19, 2007, from www.nursingadvocacy.org/media/tv/er.html

Center for Nursing Advocacy. (2006d). *What's the big deal about 'naughty nurse' images in the media? I mean, no one believes nurses really dress like that!* Retrieved February 19, 2007, from www.nursingadvocacy.org/faq/naughty_nurse.html

Center for Nursing Advocacy. (2006e). *Do physicians deliver better care than advanced practice nurses?* Retrieved February 19, 2007, from www.nursingadvocacy.org/faq/apn_md_relative_merits.html

Center for Nursing Advocacy. (2006f). *Are you sure nurses are autonomous? Based on what I've seen, it sure looks like physicians are calling the shots.* Retrieved February 25, 2007, from www.nursingadvocacy.org/faq/autonomy.html

Center for Nursing Advocacy. (2006g). *Family presence and the physician in charge.* Retrieved on February 26, 2007, from www.nursingadvocacy.org/news/2006/apr/03_new_yorker.html

Center for Nursing Advocacy. (2006h). *CVS pharmacist returns from Matrix; can now download entire nursing curriculum into your brain in four hours!* Retrieved February 19, 2007, from www.nursingadvocacy.org/news/2006/jan/24_cvs.html

Center for Nursing Advocacy. (2006i). *Touching the world.* Retrieved February 19, 2007, from www.nursingadvocacy.org/media/commercials/jnj_2005.html

Center for Nursing Advocacy. (2006j). *Response from Johnson & Johnson.* Retrieved February 14, 2007, from www.nursingadvocacy.org/media/commercials/jnj_2005_response.html

Center for Nursing Advocacy. (2006k). *But when I became a physician, I put away nursing things.* Retrieved February 19, 2007, from www.nursingadvocacy.org/news/2006/jul/08_houston_chron.html

Center for Nursing Advocacy. (2006l). *Debugging the "electronic nurse."* Retrieved February 19, 2007, from www.nursingadvocacy.org/news/2006/sep/20_electronic_nurse.html

Center for Nursing Advocacy. (2007a). *Annual Golden Lamp Awards—Best media depictions of nursing.* Retrieved February 14, 2007, from www.nursingadvocacy.org/press/releases/golden/lamp_awards.html

Center for Nursing Advocacy. (2007b). *News on nursing in the media.* Retrieved on February 26, 2007, from www.nursingadvocacy.org/news/news.html

Center for Nursing Advocacy. (2007c). The work of Beatrice Kalisch and Philip Kalisch on nursing's public image and the nursing shortage. Retrieved May 8, 2007, from www.nursingadvocacy.org/research/lit/kalisch_kalisch.html

Darbyshire, P., & Gordon, S. (2005). Exploring popular images and reputations of nurses and nursing. In J. Daly, et al. (Eds.). *Professional nursing: Concepts, issues, and challenges.* (pp. 69–92). New York: Springer Publishing Company.

Freed, J. (2006). *Model of the communication cycle: Communication creates reality.* Retrieved February 11, 2007 from www.media-visions.com/communication.html

Glik, D. C. (2003). *Health communication in popular media formats.* American Public Health Association Annual Meeting presentation. Retrieved February 11, 2007, from www.medscape.com/viewarticle/466709

Henry J. Kaiser Family Foundation (2004). *Entertainment education and health in the United States.* Retrieved February 19, 2007, from www.kff.org/entmedia/7047.cfm

Henry J. Kaiser Family Foundation. (2003). *Survey of ER viewers: Summary of results.* Retrieved February 19, 2007, from www.kff.org/womenshealth/1358-ers.cfm

Henry J. Kaiser Family Foundation. (2002). *The impact of TV's health content: A case study of ER viewers.* Retrieved February 19, 2007, from www.kff.org/entmedia/3230-index.cfm

HHS Press Office. (2004). HHS Secretary Tommy G. Thompson launches third annual "take a loved one to the doctor day." Retrieved February 15, 2007, from www.blackamericaweb.com/site.aspx/health/drday/drdayrel

JWT Communications. (2000). *Memo to nurses for a healthier tomorrow coalition members on a focus group study of 1800 school children in 10 U.S. cities.* Retrieved February 19, 2007, from www.nursingadvocacy.org/research/lit/jwt_memo1.html

Kalisch, P. A., & Kalisch, B. J. (1986). A comparative analysis of nurse and physician characters in the entertainment media. *Journal of Advanced Nursing*, 11(2), 179–195.

Lewenson, S. B. (1993). *Taking charge: Nursing, suffrage, and feminism in America, 1873–1920.* New York: Garland Press.

Mason, D. J., Dodd, C. J., & Glickstein, B. (2007). Harnessing the power of the media to influence health policy and politics. In D. J. Mason, J. K. Leavitt, & M. W. Chafee (Eds.), *Policy and politics in nursing and health care* (5th ed.). (pp. 149–168). St. Louis, MO: Saunders Elsevier.

Mason, D. J., Leavitt, J. K., & Chafee, M. W. (Eds.). (2007). *Policy and politics in nursing and health care*, 5th ed. St. Louis, MO: Saunders Elsevier.

Nelson, S., & Gordon, S. (2006). *The complexities of care: Nursing reconsidered.* Ithaca, NY: Cornell University Press.

Newspaper Association of America Foundation. (2005). *Speaking of a free press: 200 years of notable quotations about press freedoms*, p. 3. Retrieved February 23, 2007, from www.naafoundation.org/pdf/Speaking_of_a_Free_Press.pdf

Pew Internet & American Life Project. (2003). *Internet health resources.* Retrieved February 23, 2007, from www.pewinternet.org/PPF/r/95/report_display.asp

Reynolds, K. (1997). *What is the transmission model of interpersonal communication and what is wrong with it?* Student paper from the University of Wales, Aberystwyth. Retrieved February 11, 2007, from www.aber.ac.uk/media/Students/kjr9601.html

Saad, L. (2006). *Gallup Poll news service: Nurses top list of most honest and ethical professions: Integrity of most medical professionals also highly rated.* Retrieved February 25, 2007, from www.galluppoll.com/content/default.aspx?ci=25888&VERSION=p

Turow, J., & Gans, R. (2002). *As seen on TV: Health policy issues in TV's medical dramas.* Report to the Henry J. Kaiser Family Foundation, p. 1. Retrieved February 11, 2007, from www.kff.org/entmedia/3231-index.cfm

U.S. Census Bureau. (2007). *Statistical abstract of the United States.* Section 24. "Media Usage and Consumer Spending: 2000 to 2009," Table 1110. Retrieved February 1, 2007, from www.census.gov/prod/2006pubs/07statab/infocomm.pdf

U.S. Department of Health and Human Services, Health Resources and Service Administration, Bureau of Health Professions, Division of Nursing. (2000). *The registered nurse population: Findings from the national sample survey of registered nurses.* Retrieved July 20, 2007, from http://bhpr.hrsa.gov/healthworkforce/reports/rnsurvey/rnss1.htm

Young, R. (2006). "Google . . . the OS for advertising." Retrieved February 11, 2007, from http://gigaom.com/2006/11/09/google-the-os-for-advertising

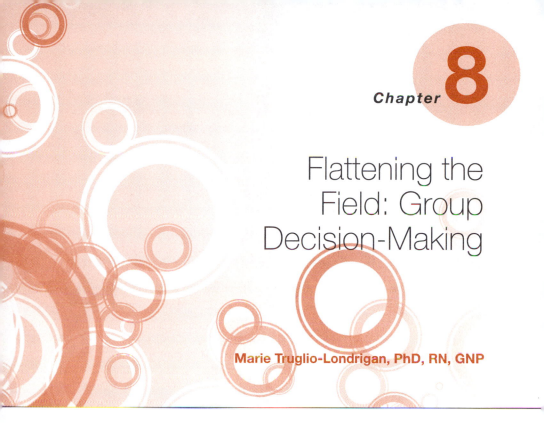

Chapter 8

Flattening the Field: Group Decision-Making

Marie Truglio-Londrigan, PhD, RN, GNP

The complexities of the U.S. health care system warrant an approach to clinical practice, education, and research that is inclusive of all disciplines and the populations that these disciplines serve. Individual practitioners, educators, and researchers find themselves making clinical decisions at the point of service throughout their daily practice. These same practitioners also find that working together in groups is essential to their practice as they attempt to meet the complex challenges that are an ever-increasing reality. These challenges include the rise of mental health issues and chronic illnesses, violence, infectious diseases, weak public health infrastructure, disaster management, threats of bioterrorism, technology, fragmented health care, and the realities of a limited pool of resources including financial and people power as evidenced by a continual struggle to maintain a sustainable nursing work force. Bruce and McKane (2000) discuss the importance of communities, health practitioners, and academicians working together in partnerships to meet these challenges. This coming *together* to work *together* brings the notion of making decisions *together*. Group decision-making, therefore, allows individuals to come together in a partnership to work toward a goal and ultimately achieve their vision. Similarly, when organizations come together to form coalitions in a partnership model, group decision-making provides the means in which the organizations can achieve its goals. Group decision-making and the process of group decision-making is an important one for nurses to learn and use in the health care settings in which they work.

What Is Group Decision-Making?

Some individuals propose that when working together in groups the decision-making process yields better decisions especially when all of the individuals have input in the process (Yoder-Wise, 2003). Groups provide for more and varied input and generate more of a commitment (Sullivan & Decker, 2005). Groups may take many forms in the health care and academic systems. For the purpose of this chapter, however, group decision-making will be discussed in relation to a group of organizations or agencies that are working together in a coalition partnership model. A *coalition* is two or more organizations coming together that join forces and share resources so that a shared concern is challenged and resolved (Sullivan, 1998). This coalition (**Table 8-1**) represents a process strategy for encouraging collaborative problem solving particularly in community settings (Kaye & Wolff, 2002). Those organizations that come together work together in a collaborative way. This collaboration is defined as "a dynamic transforming process of creating a power sharing partnership for pervasive application in health care practice, education, research, and organizational settings for the purposeful attention to needs and problems in order to achieve likely successful outcomes. . ." (Sullivan, 1998, p. 6).

Reflecting on the definition just given, several characteristics clearly are evident. These include a dynamic transforming process, power-sharing partnerships, attention to needs and problems, and successful outcomes. Inherent in these characteristics are the important concepts of relationships, trust, and group decision-making. In order for there to be a power-sharing partnership, some type of relationship must be evident. Initially, the partnership is held together because of the vision that may have brought the group together. For example, a community coalition may consist of several health, educational, and social organizations of a local town to plan and build a skate park for its young residents. This skate park may be used by skateboarders and in-liners who are usually a particular aggregate of the preteen and teen population in a given community. Early in the development of the coalition, the partnership and the relationship between and among all of the organiza-

Table 8-1

Visual Depiction of the Steps of a Coalition

Need present in the community

Need identified by a lead organization based on data collected via
subjective and objective evidence

Lead organization has a vision pertaining to the need

Lead organization conducts an assessment of the community
to determine other organizations or agencies that may have
shared values and beliefs and thus display an interest in the
presenting need

Lead organization reaches out to these other organizations or
agencies and introduces the need and vision

Community organizations or agencies who share similar values
and beliefs may have a desire to work with the lead organization
on the identified issue and agree to be a member of the coalition
thus establishing the beginning partnerships

The structure of the coalition is developed as well as the
processes needed to ensure communication, shared work, shared
problem solving, shared goal setting, all being facilitated due to a
shared decision-making and the development of trust with time

Coalition partners identify with key informants from the community
plans, implementation strategies, and evaluation components
based in best practice

Coalition partners share in the work or implementation of the plan

Outcomes noted and documented

tions is held together by their vision: In this case, the vision is the need for a safe environment for its young residents so that they may practice their sport in a safe manner.

The relationships that take form in the development of the coalition reflect a complex network of connections that sets the stage for the development of trust. As the coalition works together, over time, affirming their relationship trust is established. With this relationship building, connection, and the development of trust, communication takes place.

Kang (1997) notes that trusting relationships facilitate efficiency and fidelity in communication and the diffusion of information. Similarly, Cartwright and Limandri (1997) note that trust is essential for open expression of views and opinions. The building of a trusting relationship within the partnerships of the coalition facilitates the coalition's ability to communicate and make decisions together or to engage in the group decision-making process. This trust is essential because without it, the coalition will not be a success. The primary reason for an unsuccessful ending is the inability of the coalition to share not only in the work but the group decision-making so necessary for a coalition's survival.

The Common Good

The overriding vision of the coalition serves as the driving force. The key term here is *overriding*. In other words, when the individual members of the coalition make formal or informal agreements to come together with the expressed purpose to work toward the vision, there is a common ground that has been established for the achievement of the common good. This shared vision leads to a shared mission and goals. It is the idea of working together for the common good that keeps the coalition vital as the partners share together in the work and decision-making. The shared vision is the driving force, the engine, that supports the activities of the coalition including shared work, shared problem solving, shared responsibility, shared goal setting, and shared planning throughout which shared group decision-making takes place (Sullivan, 1998). A visual representation of this is noted in **Figure 8-1**. This model is similar to the model of decision-making being put forth in this text. Every step in the process of the coalition development and in the working of the coalition toward the achievement of the vision or the mission and goals of this model is enacted because of the coalition's ability to engage in group decision-making for the common good.

Shared Values and Collective Action for the Common Good

There are many shared values and actions (**Table 8-2**) which support a coalition's work and facilitates a group's decision-making process. The overriding vision presented earlier is the core from which the mission and goals are developed. Together, the shared vision, mission, and goal are important and represent the essence of the coalition, the very being for its existence. It is this shared vision that prompts the members of the coalition to act in a collective way, to work together without thought to self-interest. It is a model of a working and trusting relationship in

Figure 8-1

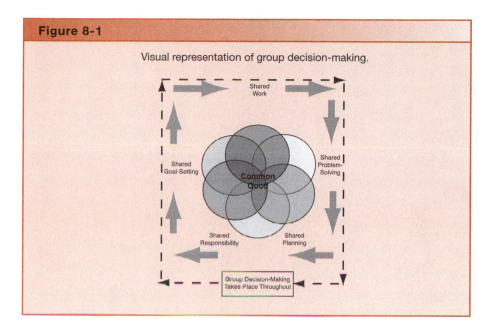

Visual representation of group decision-making.

which the common good is given precedence over the interests of the individual organizations involved. This illustrates another value of equal importance, which is that the members of a coalition need to be other centered for the support and facilitation of the common good.

In order for there to be group decision-making between and among all members of a coalition, the group decision-making process must permit "broad participation in determining the course of the coalition" (Kaye & Wolff, 2002, p. 33). The primary concern is the vision of the entire coalition; therefore, the voices of all of the members of the coalition must be heard and valued. In the group decision-making model, there is a kind of collectivism for which all of the organizations involved share in the work including the planning, task accomplishments, implementation of strategies, and evaluation of outcomes in such a way that exemplifies inclusiveness (Woehrle, 2003). A coalition is nonhierarchical. There is no "power over" in a coalition, only "power with" as the members of the coalition exemplify the values of sharing and inclusiveness for the common good. This requires equal empowerment of all members of a coalition in order for the entity to communicate and work together. Any opposition to this broad participation and inclusiveness inhibits the working of the coalition. Working with groups that also may include consumers is challenging and there always is the possibility for hierarchical relationships which may result in decisions that are not representative of the view of the entire group (Allen, Dyas, & Jones, 2004). This, however, violates the spirit of a coalition.

Table 8-2

Shared Values of Coalition Members

Shared Vision
Shared Mission/Goal
Common Good
Collectivism
Other Centeredness
Broad participation
Inclusiveness
Respect
Time
Self-Reflection
Share
Power With
Present
Attentive
Intention
Collegiality
Communication
Listen
Value Other

This highlights yet another value essential to the group decision-making process: the value of shared communication and the respect for the time necessary for this shared communication to take place. The communication exchange that takes place between and among all organizational members of the coalition must be considered and demonstrate the inclusiveness discussed earlier and engage all members' perspectives: "Exclusion generates 'we-they' dynamic. . .; What is needed is a pluralistic process . . ." (Michaels, 2002, p. 2). Part of this time is needed for self-reflection. The communication necessary for group decision-making is complex. Greitemeyer, Schulz-Hardt, Brodbeck, and Frey (2006) identify that making decisions in organizations and in life where there are groups as players in the decision-making process requires more time and effort among the people involved. Members of the coalition must consciously be present, attentive, and listen with intention in every respect. Michaels (2002) speaks to this same issue and notes that through the ". . . practice of listening, intentional speaking, and conscious self-monitoring . . ." (p. 1), the purpose of the group will be realized. There is no room for an atmosphere of competition, only collegiality and working together for the common good. Self-reflection enables members of the coalition to become involved in moments of self-checking, asking questions such as: How do I feel about what is happening?; Can I support what is happening?; Do I feel listened to?; Do I feel that what I have to say is valued?; Is the coalition taking on a task that is congruent with the original vision, mission, and goals?; Is any one member of the coalition attempting to usurp power? Answers to these questions may give clues to how one feels about the progress and process of the coalition and how one is responding or reacting to others in the coalition at any given moment in time, thus avoiding conflict.

Why Consensus?

Working in groups takes time, self-reflection, and a commitment to the greater good. There is a tremendous amount of work in setting the stage for the group to work together. A coalition for which members take the time to move together toward a common good requires a group decision-making process that facilitates broad participation that may also assist in the avoidance of conflicts. One example of a participatory group decision-making model is that of consensus. This group decision-making model is nonhierarchical; instead, decisions are made through a collective and participatory approach. Woehrle (2003) notes that "consensus is that 'general agreement' is reached" (p. 15). It is, however, the process that unfolds in the group that facilitates this "general agreement." This process illustrates "harmony, cooperation, sympathy, and group solidarity. . . . It does require people willing to find common ground in principle and practical solutions that everyone can live with (Senge, Kleiner, Roberts, Ross, Roth, & Smith, 1999, pp. 378–379). There is no vote whereby the majority "wins" and the minority "loses"; rather, the group process is such that everyone has the opportunity to participate and contribute and the outcome is a decision that everyone believes they can live with (Woehrle, 2003). Groups that make decisions using the majority rule may only "partially achieve the goals of quality and acceptance" (Yoder-Wise, 2003, p. 82) in reference to both the decision being made and the members of the coalition. Woehrle (2003) describes how in the consensus model of decision-making, it is better to hold off on a decision than to take a vote that excludes individuals: "The balancing factor in consensus is that participants hold the responsibility to 'step aside' if their concerns are not pressing enough to merit blocking the unity of the group" (p. 16). How the group accomplishes this is through the provision of time for dialogue. With time and the dialogue that unfolds, coalition members begin to see and understand what other coalition members may be speaking about and again in time these thoughts and ideas become integrated into their own. This idea is synonymous with Gadamer (1976) who spoke to the language of conversation that provides the medium for understanding as individuals use language to express themselves and listen. The outcome is consensus. As Woehrle (2003) described this experience: ". . . time is spent on the process of persuasion" (p. 4).

Techniques and Tools for Consensus

This consensus group decision-making process is not easy. The one overriding factor that is important throughout the process is that the coalition holds true to the value of the common good and the vision at hand. This is what spurs the coalition members to continue with the group process until consensus is reached. Members of the coalition may use certain techniques and tools to facilitate the storming of ideas thus contributing to the communication and the generation of alternative ideas. First and foremost, the members of the coalition need to understand group process and consensus decision-making. Living in a culture where competition and winning is a primary value will warrant time for education and a coming to understand what consensus is and how to work together in this type of model. Exercises on communication and listening skills may be necessary. Similarly, education on conduct within the group also is essential, particularly the roles inherent in the group.

Group decision-making does not mean that people just get together and speak without thought to process. In fact, the process is facilitated by the members in the group who all assume certain roles and responsibilities. AIDS Coalition to Unleash Power (2006) identifies several roles key to the process of consensus decision-making. These roles include facilitator, vibes-watcher, and recorder. Huber (2006) identifies the facilitator as the one who "conducts the meeting, ensuring that everyone has the opportunity to speak, maintains the focus of the meeting, and controls the problem participants" (p. 577). The facilitator may be the individual(s) who represents the lead organization of the coalition. This individual facilitates the process with agenda setting, getting all participants involved in the communication and in the work of the coalition, defining and redefining the vision, and works with all members of the coalition to brainstorm when it comes to making decisions or identifying alternative approaches and solutions to problem solving (Conflict Research Consortium, 1998). This brainstorming is just one technique, among many, that may be used to create an environment in which ideas are freely expressed without critique. The goal is to stimulate as many ideas as possible (Yoder-Wise, 2003). Part of the facilitator's role when generating alternatives is to work with the members of the coalition as they collectively evaluate costs and benefits as well as barriers to implementation of the alternatives discussed (Conflict Research Consortium, 2006).

In a given situation where a particular decision must be made, the facilitator, after a period of time brainstorming, assists the group in narrowing down the alternatives to one approach in the form of a proposal. It is the facilitator's responsibility to ensure that all individuals were given the time to express their own ideas and beliefs. Once the final proposal is noted and there appears to be no new ideas being generated for that proposal, the facilitator may ask if there are any objections to its implementation (AIDS Coalition to Unleash Power, 2006). If after a period of silence and there are no objections, then consensus is reached. If there are members of the coalition who cannot support the proposal, then they may express their objection. Some members of the coalition may express their objection, yet indicate that they will still abide by the proposal in the interest of the vision of the coalition. Other members of the coalition may not be able to support the proposal and may not be able to abide by the proposal on any level. In this event, the members of the coalition note this and there is a reaffirming of the vision and a return to the process.

Throughout the consensus model of the group decision-making process, two other roles, vibes-watcher and recorder, are critical to the group process. *Vibes-watcher* is a member of the coalition who works side by side with the facilitator. This individual assists the facilitator as they watch the workings of the group and comments on what they observe in terms of individual participation, communication patterns within the group, and how individuals within the group are relating—or not—to one another. The *recorder* is the individual who documents the discussions and manages the agenda and time. This role is important because the individual keeps a record of the discussion for archival purposes and for the instances when the group needs to review what discussions have been issued in the past (AIDS Coalition to Unleash Power, 2006).

Outcomes of Consensus

According to Yoder-Wise (2003), the outcomes that occur as a result of engaging the consensus model of decision-making are evident because of the different individuals and organizations involved: "... when individuals with different knowledge, skills, and resources collaborate to solve a problem or make a decision, the likelihood of a quality outcome is increased" (p. 82). The inclusiveness of the group and the participation between and among all members of the coalition creates an environment rich with diversity of opinion. These varying opinions that are brought to the group are born out of individual-rich experiences and histories. This atmosphere only serves to create an environment of growth, commitment, and innovation (Mansbridge, 2003). It makes sense, therefore, that in situations in which all individuals are directly involved in the coalition and decision-making process, there is an enhanced likelihood that decisions and the acceptance of these decisions are increased because all parties have a hand in the process and are committed to the vision. Other advantages include an increase in unity, commitment, innovation, and trust (Mansbridge, 2003).

Nurses work in groups in every practice arena and have historically done so. An understanding of group decision-making can only serve to enhance and enrich nursing practice. In addition, the outcome of a practice that applies and supports the group decision-making process demonstrates solutions that are sustainable over time. An example of this group decision-making process is noted in the following case study.

Case Study

In the northeast section of the United States, there is a town located not far from a major city. One spring, the local elementary school nurse heard the students in the elementary school complaining about the town police. Their complaint centered around one particular topic. They were skateboarders and in-line skaters with no place to practice their sport. As a result, these young teens found themselves grinding curbs and handrails anywhere possible. (*Grinding* is where the teens practice the use of their skateboards on sidewalks, curbs, and staircase railings.) More often than not, these curbs and handrails were on town property, on private property, or in parking lots. The elementary school nurse in the town spoke to the young teens and noted that the conflict that was arising centered on the fact that the police were only trying to protect these young teens and other people in the town who found themselves accosted by the fast-moving action of these young individuals practicing their sport.

The elementary school nurse was a resident of the town and decided to observe these young teens perform their sport. What the school nurse found was that indeed the practice of a much-loved sport was in evidence. With each trick on the skateboard came "whoops and hollers" from the group, supporting one another to "keep going" or to "keep trying." The school nurse also noted, that most, if not all, of the young teens were not wearing protective gear and many found themselves in the direct line of oncoming traffic. In fact, the school nurse noted that there had been a recent death in another town as a young teen skateboarded in a major parking lot. As a school nurse, health promotion and protection from injury was always in the forefront of practice. This school nurse gathered the young teens into her office and made a recommendation. "Why do you not go to the town hall and speak with the head of the recreation department? Maybe, just maybe, the town would be willing to work to build you a park." At the beginning, the young teens looked at the nurse with disbelief and asked: "How could this be? Would someone actually be willing to listen to us?"

After this initial meeting with the school nurse, the students, along with their parents, did go to the town hall to speak with the director of the department of recreation. The director was willing to listen, however, he wanted evidence that there was a need for a special park, and he wanted to see that other individuals and organizations supported such an idea. From this second meeting, it was clear to the young teens and their families that if their vision, a place to practice their sport in a safe environment, was to become a reality, they needed to contact other organizations. Parents and the young teens put their heads together and came up with a list. The school system, police department, town board leaders, department of recreation, chamber of commerce, local medical group, and the hospital were all organizations or agencies that had an interest in this particular issue.

A third meeting was called by the parents and young teens that were inclusive of all of the listed organizations. All of the organizations displayed an interest and all wanted to work together to build a skate park for this population; thus, an informal coalition was developed. Some were primarily interested in getting "the kids off of the streets" and some were interested in "protecting the young teens from injury."

The various constituents that came together shared an overriding vision, which was to build a skate park for this particular population of young teens. The lead organization was the department of recreation. This department assumed responsibility for any and all town recreation activities. An assessment of such activities revealed that indeed there were many local recreational activities—soccer, swimming, basketball, football, golf, disk golf, hockey, bowling, and tennis, just to name a few—but nothing to support the individuals who practiced skateboarding. Although there was plenty of anecdotal evidence that suggested this to be an unsafe sport if practiced outside of a designated area, there was no objective data such as number of fractures in the emergency room due to skateboarding accidents as a result of not wearing protective gear. The lead agency noted that although this would be great evidence, they were willing to support the skateboard park with the anecdotal evidence if there were enough teens who would be using the park, and if funding could be found to support this type of park.

All the members of this informal coalition took on separate distinct roles, yet each coalition member was integral to the achievement of the vision. The recreation department was the lead organization and responsible for ensuring that communication between and among all members was sustained. The facilitator of the meetings, the director of the recreation department, ensured that all members of the coalition—especially the young teens—had a say in the discussion and that all members were listened to. Meetings were held at times convenient to everyone.

During these meetings, the vision of the skateboard park remained at the forefront with the discussions centered on how to realize that vision. Several times during the planning process, the members of the coalition went to town meetings to keep the town board advised as to the process. The chamber of commerce was involved so that the town businesses were kept in the loop about the status of the park because of their hope that these young teens would eliminate their practice in the front of their stores. This involvement also was important because the business members in town also would be influential with fund-raising efforts. The hospital and the medical group provided the information pertaining to the need for such a park with particular emphasis on the health promotion and protection of this young population of teens. The school system, local elementary school nurse, and the town police supported the students in their planning and in the generation of ideas for fund-raising along with the parents. The parents and teens were responsible for heading up the fund-raising efforts as well as the planning and the building of the park. The key here was the young teens actively engaging in the planning of the park design so that they would have a hand in the selection of the pipes and ramps that they found most useful to the practice of their sport.

Key decisions made by the coalition included the need for the park, the location of the park, the equipment in the park, how to raise money for the park, how to build the park, the monitoring of the park once built, rules of conduct in the park, and fees to use the park.

As with any coalition, all members' ideas were critical to the success of the vision. In this case study, group decision-making using the consensus model was in evidence throughout. For example, when looking for an appropriate site to build the park, all members of the coalition assessed every available free space within the town. Given that there was not a tremendous amount of unused space, this presented only three options. The coalition members engaged in discussion about these three spaces under the guidance of the director of the department of recreation. Ultimately, all members respected the others and listened to alternative solutions. In the end, the proposal for one particular site was met with agreement by all members of the coalition. In the final analysis, the skateboard park was built and the use of the park by the young teens has been in strong evidence.

Conclusion

In today's health care arena, complex problems warrant the development of partnerships among multiple organizations. These multiple organizations may work together in the form of a coalition so that each may access their own strengths yet together create a front so that a common vision becomes a reality. These partnerships serve a purpose to work together to achieve a common vision, mission, and goal. Throughout the workings of the coalition partnership, group decision-making strategies such as consensus decision-making are critical. Working together and conducting themselves according to the values that serve the coalition and the achievement of the vision is the realization of the common good and the vision. Nurses can use this model in the multiple health care settings in which they work.

References

AIDS Coalition to Unleash Power [Act Up]. (n.d.). *Civil disobedience training*. Retrieved April 26, 2006, from www.actupny.org/documents/CDdocuments/Consensus.html

Allen, J., Dyas, J., & Jones, M. (2004). Building consensus in health care: A guide to using the nominal group technique. *British Journal of Community Nursing, 9*(3), 110–114.

Bruce, R. A., & McKane, S. U. (Eds.). (2000). *Community-based public health: A partnership model*. Washington, DC: American Public Health Association.

Cartwright, J., & Limandri, B. (1997). The challenge of multiple roles in the qualitative clinician research-participant client relationship. *Qualitative Health Research, 7*(2), 223–235.

Conflict Research Consortium. (1998). *International online training program on intractable conflict: Consensus building*. Retrieved April 28, 2006, from www.colorado.edu/conflict/peace/treatment/consens.htm

Gadamer, H. G. (1976). *Philosophical hermeneutics* (D. Linge, Trans. & Ed.). Los Angeles: University of California Press.

Greitemeyer, T., Schulz-Hardt, S., Brodbeck, F., & Frey, D. (2006). Information sampling and group decision-making: The effects of an advocacy decision procedure and task experience. *Journal of Experimental Psychology: Applied, 22*(1), 31–42.

Huber, D. (2006). *Leadership and nursing care management*. Philadelphia: Saunders Elsevier.

Kang, R. (1997). Building community capacity for health promotion: A challenge for public health nurses. In B. W. Spradley & J. A. Allender (Eds.), *Readings in community health nursing* (pp. 221–241). New York: Lippincott.

Kaye, G., & Wolff, T. (Eds.). (2002). *From the ground up: A workbook on coalition building & community development*. Amherst, MA: AHEC/Community Partners, Inc.

Mansbridge, J. (2003). Consensus in context: A guide for social movements. In P. G. Coy (Ed.), *Consensus Decision Making, Northern Ireland and Indigenous Movements* (Vol. 24, pp. 229–253). St. Louis, MO: Elsevier Science Ltd.

Michaels, C. L. (2002). Circle communication: An old form of communication useful for 21st century leadership. Nursing Administration Quarterly, 26(5), 1–10.

Senge, R., Kleiner, A., Roberts, C., Ross, R., Roth, G., & Smith, B. (1999). The dance of change: The challenges to sustaining momentum in learning organizations. New York: Doubleday.

Sullivan, E. J., & Decker, P. J. (2005). Effective leadership and management in nursing. Upper Saddle River, NJ: Prentice Hall.

Sullivan, T. (1998). Collaboration: A health care imperative. New York: McGraw-Hill.

Woehrle, L. M. (2003). Claims-making and consensus in collective group processes. In P. G. Coy (Ed.), Consensus decision-making, Northern Ireland and indigenous movements (Vol. 24, pp. 3–30). St. Louis, MO: Elsevier Science Ltd.

Yoder-Wise, P. S. (2003). Leading and managing in nursing. St. Louis, MO: Mosby.

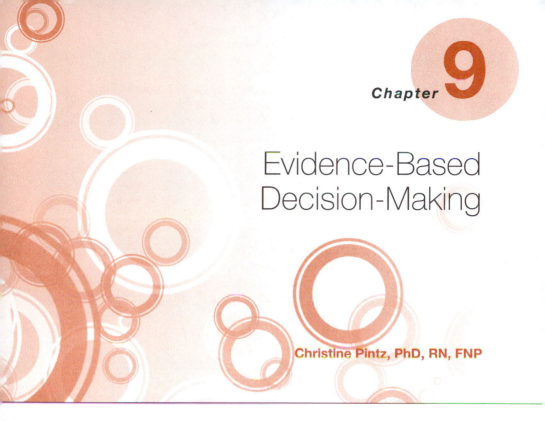

Christine Pintz, PhD, RN, FNP

Chapter 9

Evidence-Based Decision-Making

Previous chapters have examined the decision-making process from various perspectives; this chapter focuses on how research-based evidence supports decision-making. Making clinical decisions entails the application of theoretical knowledge and research to clinical situations (Rashotte & Carnevale, 2004). Health care practitioners are taught to make clinically sound decisions. Typically, their decisions are based on the knowledge attained during professional training combined with clinical experience, both in school and after. Although experience is an important component of the decision-making process, there is growing support in the health professions for combining the clinician's knowledge and clinical experience with current research-based evidence. Clinical decisions are often made under uncertainty, but the extent of uncertainty diminishes when relevant and valid evidence is available to support those decisions (McNeil, 2001).

Keeping abreast of current research can be a daunting task for busy clinicians; there seems to be a limitless amount of information that is continually updated. Straus and Sackett (1997) argue that evidence-based practice (EBP) approaches can assist in the management of this large volume of information. They maintain that EBP helps clinicians ask clinically pertinent questions, provides a framework for evaluating research, and encourages clinicians to incorporate research with clinical expertise.

EBP is not a new concept. Clinical practices should be derived from evidence based on well-designed and well-implemented research. Guyatt and colleagues (2000) maintain that intuition, unsystematic clinical experience and pathophysiological rationale are insufficient parameters for making clinical decisions. Clinical decisions should be based on the examination of clinical research. The use of EBP expands the decision-making process because it involves applying research to clinical practice. EBP employs a systematic approach to analyzing the best research, synthesizing it, judging whether it is clinically relevant and then applying it to practice. Ultimately, the goal of EBP is to translate research into practice.

The Evidence-Based Practice Trend

The trend toward EBP began with Archie Cochrane, a British epidemiologist. Cochrane published a book criticizing the medical profession for not providing critiques of research so policy makers and organizations could make sound decisions about health care. He advocated for the use of evidence from randomized controlled trials (RCTs) that would provide more scientifically valid information than other sources of evidence. Because of his influence, the Cochrane Collaboration was established to develop, maintain, and update systematic clinical reviews of research (Fineout-Overholt, Melnyk, & Schultz, 2005). A working group at McMaster University published an article advocating the use of research in teaching medical students and originated the phrase evidence-based medicine (White, 2004).

The terms evidence-based medicine, evidence-based nursing, or perhaps a more inclusive term, evidence-based practice have a number of definitions. Sackett and colleagues (1996) maintain that it is the "conscientious, explicit, and judicious use of current best evidence in making decisions about the care of individual patients." However, evidence from systematic research is not enough. Fineout-Overholt, Melnyk, and Shultz (2005) refer to EBP as a problem-solving approach to clinical care that integrates the conscientious use of evidence from "well-designed studies, the clinician's expertise and the patient's values and preferences" (p. 335). Their definition includes patient preferences and the application of the clinician's expertise as essential to making the best clinical decisions. Moreover, Guyatt and Rennie (2002) maintain that evidence alone is insufficient for making clinical decisions and that clinical decisions should be based on the comparison of the benefits and risks, patient inconvenience, and costs combined with a consideration of the patient's values.

Why Evidence-Based Practice?

The purpose of EBP is to assist clinicians in making clinical decisions that are associated with the best patient outcomes. Experienced clinicians often employ *heuristics* (experience-based knowledge) in order to make decisions. While using heuristics often leads to rapid problem-solving, they may be associated with biased thinking that leads to error. To counter these biases, clinicians are urged to develop decisions based on fact or "evidence." Patient outcomes are better when clinical care is based on relevant and valid research and not on outdated information or interventions (McNeil, 2001). However, the role of EBP in promoting better health care outcomes is only beginning to be realized (Clancy, Slutsky, & Patton, 2004).

The practice of EBP involves engaging in a systematic process of finding and utilizing the best evidence to support clinical practices. Straus and Sackett (1997) describe the process of EBP as involving five steps. When employing the EBP process the clinician should:

1. Ask a clinically focused and relevant question.
2. Efficiently identify the best evidence with which to answer the question.
3. Critically appraise the evidence for validity and clinical usefulness.
4. Apply the results to clinical practice.
5. Evaluate performance of the evidence in the clinical application.

These steps can help guide the clinician through the evidence-based process. By following these steps, the clinician can form answerable questions and by identifying evidence, they can find support to base their decisions.

Asking a Clinical Question

Asking a clinically focused question can assist in the development of questions that guide the literature search. A good clinical question focuses on how to improve the care of a particular patient. In contrast, a research question generates knowledge that is generalizable to a population and guides practice from a broader perspective (Fineout-Overholt et al., 2005). One way to formulate a pertinent clinical question is to use the P.I.C.O. model for clinical questions. In the P.I.C.O. format, "P" stands for patient population; "I" stands for the intervention; "C" for comparison or what are alternative interventions; and "O" is for outcomes (Weinfield & Finkelstein, 2005).

Where to Find Evidence to Guide Practice

Sources of clinically based evidence have increased in the last few years so that clinicians can more readily find resources to enhance their practice. There are a number of sources of appraised and synthesized research. This approach relies on experts to take on the complex and time-consuming task of sorting through the literature and finding clinically relevant and valid studies. Search engines of literature databases allow clinicians to search the literature to answer particular questions (White, 2004).

There are a number of resources for already summarized and evaluated research; for instance, the Cochrane Library that is sponsored by the Cochrane Collection. The Cochrane Library consists of systematic review databases. Fifty collaborative review groups contribute systematic reviews that focus on specific clinical questions. "Patient-oriented evidence that matters" (POEMs) are another set of tools that allow clinicians to focus on what is important rather than on all available literature. POEMs are published in many journals such as *American Family Physician* and the *British Medical Journal* (White, 2004).

Additionally, there are many databases that allow clinicians to search the literature for their own questions. The CINAHL database includes all aspects of nursing, allied health, and alternative health and community medicine. The CINAHL database indexes 1,200 journals, with more than one third in the field of nursing. The MEDLINE database is produced by the National Library of Medicine (NLM). It has more than 10 million records and indexes more than 4,800 journals. There is free access through the NLM's site PubMed. The PsychInfo database is produced by the American Psychological Association. All areas of psychology and its application to other fields of study are included (Klem & Weiss, 2005; Morrisey & DeBourgh, 2001).

These resources can help clinicians by using "just-in-time" strategies for the management of large volumes of information. Just in time refers to the focus of efforts to increase efficiency, productivity, motivation, and waste reduction (White, 2006). One way of minimizing waste is to reduce the time it takes to identify evidence-based resources. By focusing information gathering to what is needed for a specific time and question, clinicians reduce wasted time. In fact, Slawson and Shaughnessy (2005) propose that instead of using information that clinicians have at hand—which often may be of poor quality (using outdated textbooks and journals, for example), clinicians should use information tools, such as decision support tools, clinical awareness systems, (i.e., *Journal Watch* or e-mail alerts) and search engines. **Table 9-1** illustrates a selection of evidence-based resources.

Assessing the Quality of Studies

Guidelines have been developed to help clinicians critically appraise the quality of studies. Assessing the quality of studies is based on a number of criteria. The Agency for Healthcare Research and Quality (2002) evaluated systems to rate the strength of scientific evidence that includes three domains. These domains help clinicians or policy makers determine whether a body of research provides information to change practice and policy. The quality rating indicates the extent to which bias is minimized for individual studies. Quantity looks at the magnitude of effect, numbers of studies, and the sample size or power. Consistency refers to whether similar findings have been reported with similar and with different study designs.

Table 9-1

Selected Evidence-Based Practice Resources

Evidence-Based Practice Resources

Agency for Healthcare Quality
http://www.ahrq.gov

The Centre for Evidence-Based Medicine
http://www.cebm.utoronto.ca

Clinical Evidence
http://www.clinicalevidence.org/ceweb/conditions/index.jsp

Cochrane Collaboration
http://www.cochrane.org

Evidence-based Nursing
http://ebn.bmjjournals.com

FIRST Consult
http://www.firstconsult.com

InfoRetriever and Daily POEMs
http://www.infopoems.com

National Guideline Clearing House
http://www.guideline.gov

Oxford Centre for Evidence-based Medicine
http://www.cebm.net

PubMed
http://www.pubmed.gov

TRIP Database (Turning Research into Practice)
http://www.tripdatabase.com

UpToDate
http://www.uptodate.com

U.S. Preventive Services Task Force
http://www.ahrq.gov/clinic/prevenix.htm

Worldviews on Evidence-Based Nursing
http://www.blackwellpublishing.com/submit.asp?ref=1545-102X&site=1

Critical Appraisal

Critical appraisal is the process of making a decision about whether a study can help to answer a clinical question. When critically appraising literature, there are three questions to ask about any kind of research: (1) Are the results valid? (2) Are they reliable, and (3) Do they apply to patient care? (Oxman, Sackett, & Guyatt, 1993). The validity refers to whether the study results were obtained through rigorous scientific methods that minimize bias and confounding variables, permitting a high level of support for an inference. Reliability pertains to the consistency and repeatability of findings across studies (Shadish, Cook, & Campbell, 2002). Lastly, in order to transfer clinical research to patient care, the study must apply to patient care.

Hierarchy of Evidence

Research designs can be arranged in a hierarchical fashion based on their ability to control for error and to support a cause-and-effect relationship. **Table 9-2** depicts study designs that make up the hierarchy.

Table 9-2	
Hierarchy of Evidence	
Research Design	
Meta-analysis	Meta-analysis is a type of systematic review that combines data from different studies. It is used to determine effective treatments and plan further research.
Systematic Reviews	Systematic reviews summarize research that addresses similar research questions. Reviews employ a systematic search and a critical appraisal of the literature.
Randomized Controlled Trial (RCT)	A randomized controlled trial is an experiment where individuals are randomly assigned into intervention or control groups.
Cohort Studies	Cohort studies follow groups of exposed and unexposed individuals who are followed up for specific outcomes. They can be prospective or retrospective.
Case Control Studies	Case control studies are studies in which patients with a condition are compared to those who do not have the condition.
Case Reports	Information based on the report of one case. Often the case describes the treatment of a rare condition.
Expert Opinion	Information based on the opinion of experts in the field.

At the top of the hierarchy are meta-analyses and systematic reviews that synthesize several studies to determine an overall effect. The next level includes experimental designs or randomized controlled trials. Cohort and case-control trials involve following a group over time either prospectively or retrospectively. The last level entails the consideration of anecdotal findings such as case studies or expert opinion. This hierarchy has prompted controversy about the kind of evidence that is relevant to practice. For example, randomized control trials often restrict the kind of patients recruited, whereas cohort studies may better reflect normal patterns of patient management. Because of the influence of bias, cohort studies may be less helpful in establishing causality.

The term *levels of evidence* refers to systems of classifying research evidence for scientific rigor and quality. Numerous examples of hierarchies exist. Most of the hierarchies are centered on the magnitude of effect sizes (as in meta-analysis), sample size, randomization, blinding, and Type I and II error rates.

Decision Analysis

Decision analysis refers to a method of analyzing decisions under conditions of uncertainty. It can help to improve decision-making when there is incomplete evidence to make the decision. Clinicians can compare the expected consequences of different management strategies. The process of decision analysis makes all the elements of the decision, so they can be modified. Although decision analysis cannot resolve all clinical controversies where clinical trial data is unavailable, it can convey important information about an intervention for a specific clinical problem. Decision analysis can examine whether a treatment is beneficial, it can consider whether there is a likely benefit, and it can identify whether there are gaps in the evidence (Ramsey, 1999).

Using Evidence for Practice

It takes many years to translate research findings into clinical practice. Many organizations and federal agencies are placing an emphasis on accelerating the translation of research to practice (Clancy et al., 2004). There are a number of methods to facilitate the transfer of research into clinical practice. The next section will focus on some of these.

Clinical Practice Guidelines

Clinical practice guidelines are quality-improving strategies that promote best practices. They help clinicians by bringing together the evidence and knowledge for decision-making about a specific health condition. According to Sackett et al. (1996), good clinical guidelines have three properties. First, they characterize practice questions and identify the decision options and outcomes. Second, they identify, evaluate, and summarize in a format that is most relevant to decision-makers. Third, they identify the decision points where evidence should be integrated with clinical experience in making decisions. Therefore, they identify the range of potential decisions and provide the evidence which, when added to individual clinical judgment and the patient's values and expectations, will help in determining and making the best decision for the patient (Sackett, Straus, Richardson, Rosenberg, & Haynes, 2000).

Should clinicians adopt a particular clinical practice guideline? Before incorporating a set of guidelines into clinical practice, the clinician should ascertain whether the guideline is valid, whether it is useful, and whether it should be applied to practice.

Guideline Development

There are three main methods of developing guidelines.

1. Evidence-based guidelines describe the strength of the evidence and try to separate opinion from evidence.
2. Consensus guidelines are the most common method of guideline development, also known as global subjective agreement of experts. Consensus guidelines should not be used because the consensus guideline is founded on expert opinion and experts can be wrong.
3. The expert opinion guideline methodology teaches clinicians to rely on experts, not empirical findings. The expert opinion guideline does not distinguish between clinical questions for which data are available and clinical questions for which no data are available (Graham & Harrison, 2005; Guyatt et al., 2006).

The American College of Chest Physicians (ACCP) created a working group to define the criteria for the optimal grading system. They also described factors that panels should consider when deciding a recommendation is weak or strong. Some factors include the quality of evidence, the importance of the outcome, the magnitude of the treatment effect, risks and burdens of the therapy, costs, and patient values. Guideline panels should make recommendations by balancing of factors such benefit, risk, burden, and cost with the quality of evidence (GRADE Working Group, 2004; Guyatt et al., 2006).

Clinical Pathways

Clinical pathways, also known as *critical pathways* or *care paths*, are multidisciplinary plans of best clinical practice. Clinical pathways differ from practice guidelines, protocols, and algorithms because they are utilized by a multidisciplinary team and have a focus on the quality and coordination of care. Clinical pathways are a distinct tool that details processes of care and highlights inefficiencies of care. Characteristics of clinical pathways include clear goals and elements of care based on evidence, best practice, and patient expectations. They also include the facilitation of communication, coordination of roles, and sequencing the activities of the multidisciplinary care team, patients, and their relatives. Additionally, clinical pathways include the documentation, monitoring, and evaluation of variances and outcomes and the identification of the appropriate resources. Care pathways enhance health care quality by improving patient outcomes, patient satisfaction, patient safety, and resource use (Every, Hochman, Becker, Kopecky, & Cannon, 2000; Pearson, Goulart-Fisher, & Lee, 1995).

Barriers to Evidence-Based Practice

Barriers may prevent the incorporation of EBP. An EBP culture may be difficult to establish because clinicians may lack the ability to identify, obtain, and critically evaluate information. Additionally, the time pressures of clinical practice and organizational barriers may diminish the application of evidence in clinical practice. Tanner, Pierce, and Pravikoff (2004) surveyed registered nurses in the United States to ascertain whether nurses were aware of the need for research-based information, if they had the ability to find resources, and if the resources were available. Their findings indicated that nurses were aware of the need for research-based information, however, they lacked the knowledge to locate these sources of information and the resources were not available. Most of the nurses participating in this study were not in the habit of reading research and did not have the ability to evaluate the research. With the potential for EBP to improve the quality of health care delivery, it is important that clinicians adopt EBP to promote best practices and avoid variations in care that can lead to errors (Stevens & Staley, 2006). Changing the organizational culture to encourage the integration of EBP requires administrative support. Support for EBP must focus not only on its importance to improving health care quality but to creating an environment of inquiry and openness to foster utilization of EBP. Strategies may include EBP committees, journal clubs, clinical coaching, or collaboration between health professional students and faculty and clinical staff (Pravikoff, 2006).

Models of Evidence-Based Practice

Several models of EBP have evolved in nursing to assist in the promotion of EBP. Some of the models involve the use of mentorship while others focus on utilizing the process of EBP as a way to advance EBP. Health care professionals and organizations can use models to help with the implementation of EBP.

Mentorship Models

The advancing research and clinical practice through close collaboration (ARCC) model is a model that provides a framework for advancing EBP within health care organizations. An EBP mentor, an advanced practice nurse, provides EBP mentorship and helps to facilitate improvements in clinical care and patient outcomes through implementation of EBP and outcomes management projects (Melnyk & Fineout-Overholt, 2005).

The clinical scholar model (Schultz, 2005) uses mentors to act as a resource to staff nurses. These mentors or clinical scholars provide the mechanism for the dissemination and creation of an EBP environment. The role is to challenge nursing practices through inquiry observation analysis and synthesis of data and application of the synthesized evidence (Fineout-Overholt, Melnyk, & Shultz, 2005).

Process Models

The Conduct and Utilization of Research in Nursing (CURN) project developed and tested a model for using research-based information in clinical settings. Research utilization is an organizational process. Planned change is integrated throughout the research utilization process and systems change is essential to establishing research-based practice on a large scale (Fineout-Overholt, Melnyk, & Schultz, 2005).

The Stetler model of research utilization (Stetler, 2001) applies research findings at the individual practitioner level. The model has six phases: (1) preparation, (2) validation, (3) comparative evaluation, (4) decision-making, (5) translation and application, and (6) evaluation. Critical thinking and decision-making are essential to this model.

The Iowa model of research in practice (Titler et al., 1994) emphasizes the translation of research into practice to improve the quality of care, and was developed from the quality assurance model using research (QAMUR). As with the CURN model, research utilization is an organizational process. Planned change principles are incorporated into research and practice. This model combines EBP with an interdisciplinary team approach.

Case Study

Evidence-based clinical guidelines provide clinicians with a way of applying evidence to specific clinical situations. This case study applies guidelines published in the 2002 National Asthma Education and Prevention Program (NAEPP) Expert Panel Report 2.

A nurse practitioner sees Jenny, an 8-year-old who is being seen for a follow-up visit because of her breathing problems. She has a history of asthma that has been well controlled until last month. Her parents took Jenny to an urgent care center 2 days ago. For the past month, she has awakened three to four times a night due to coughing. Her mother has noticed that Jenny has had trouble breathing a few times when she is running outside. She was treated at the urgent care center with nebulized albuterol and her wheezing completely resolved. She was not given steroids. In addition, her peak flow values, which were 70 percent of normal upon admission to urgent care, increased to 80 percent after treatment. Today, her peak flow is 80 percent of normal and she is not wheezing. Her family recently adopted a cat.

The nurse practitioner uses the NAEPP *Guidelines for the Diagnosis and Management of Asthma* (2002) to treat her patients with asthma. These guidelines are based on synthesized reviews of the literature and recommendations for practice are made by an expert panel who review the research and update recommendations. These guidelines guide practice related to the use of medications, of monitoring and prevention of asthma. According to the NAEPP asthma guidelines, it is important to determine the patient's asthma severity level in order to target treatment based on the guidelines. Jenny's symptoms are consistent with mild persistent asthma because her forced expiratory volume is 80 percent and her symptoms were present only a few times last month and less than once a week at night. Because she has mild persistent asthma, the treatment that corresponds to this level consists of using a daily low-dose steroid inhaler. Patient education that is especially important for this patient consists of a review of medications and self-monitoring, identification of asthma triggers, presence of an action plan, and a review of the use of inhaler, spacer, and peak-flow meter. Lastly, it is important to determine whether Jenny will require referral for specialty care. According to the guidelines, mild persistent asthma can be treated by a primary care practitioner and does not require referral for specialty care.

Conclusion

Clinical decisions about patient care should be based on the best re-search evidence. The best research evidence refers to methodologically sound and clinically relevant research that incorporates the cost, safety, and effectiveness of interventions with risks and benefits and patient perspectives (DiCenso, 2003). EBP offers a systematic framework and set of tools for making decisions. By implementing the process of EBP, individual clinicians as well as institutions foster an EBP environment that has the potential to improve patient care.

References

Agency for Healthcare Research and Quality. (2002). *Systems to rate the strength of scientific evidence* (AHRQ Publication No. 02-E015). Retrieved September 15, 2006, from www.ahrq.gov/clinic/epcsums/strengthsum.pdf

Clancy, C. M., Slutsky, J. R., & Patton, L. T. (2004). Evidence-based health care 2004: AHRQ moves research to translation and implementation. *Health Services Research, 39,* xv–xxiii.

DiCenso, A. (2003). Evidence-based nursing practice: How to get there from here. *Nursing Leadership, 16,* 20–26.

Every, N. R., Hochman, J., Becker, R., Kopecky, S., & Cannon, C. P. (2000). Critical pathways: A review. *Circulation, 101,* 461–465.

Fineout-Overholt, E., Melnyk, B. M., & Schultz, A. (2005). Transforming health care from the inside out: Advancing evidence-based practice in the 21st century. *Journal of Professional Nursing, 21,* 335–344.

GRADE Working Group. (2004). Grading quality of evidence and strength of recommendations. *British Medical Journal, 328,* 1482–1486.

Graham, I. D., & Harrison, M. B. (2005). Evaluation and adaptation of clini-cal practice guidelines. *Evidence Based Nursing, 8,* 68–72.

Guyatt, G., & Rennie, D. (2002). *Users' guide to the medical literature: Essentials of evidence-based practice.* Chicago: AMA Press.

Guyatt, G., Gutterman, D., Baumann, M. H., Addrizzo-Harris, D., Hylek, E. M., Phillips, B., Raskob, G., Lewis, S. Z., & Schunemann, H. (2006). Grading strength of recommendations and quality of evidence in clini-cal guidelines. *CHEST, 129,* 174–181.

Guyatt, G., Haynes, R. B., Jaeschke, R. Z., Cook, D. J., Green, L., Naylor, C. D., Wilson, M.C., & Richardson, W. S., for the Evidence-Based Medicine Working Group. (2000). Evidence-based medicine: Principles for ap-plying the user's guide to patient care. *Journal of the American Medical Association, 284,* 1290–1296.

Klem, M. L., & Weiss, P. M. (2005). Evidence-based resources and the role of librarians in developing evidence-based practice curricula. *Journal of Professional Nursing, 21,* 380–387.

McNeil, B. J. (2001). Hidden barriers to improvements in the quality of care. *New England Journal of Medicine, 345,* 12–20.

Melnyk, B. M., & Fineout-Overholt, E. (2005). *Evidence-based practice in nursing & healthcare: A guide to best practice.* Philadelphia: Lippincott Williams & Wilkins.

Morrisey, L. L., & DeBourgh, G. A. (2001). Finding evidence: Refining literature searching skills for the advanced practice nurse. *AACN Clinical Issues, 12,* 560–577.

National Asthma Education and Prevention Program. (2002). *Guidelines for the diagnosis and management of asthma—Update on selected topics 2002.* (NIH Publication No. 97-4051). Retrieved August 20, 2006, from www.nhlbi.nih.gov/health/prof/lung/index.htm#asthma

Oxman, A. D., Sackett, D. L., & Guyatt, G. H. (1993). Users' guides to the medical literature. I. How to get started. The Evidence-Based Medicine Working Group. *Journal of the American Medical Association, 270,* 2093–2095.

Pearson, S. D., Goulart-Fisher, D., & Lee, T. H. (1995). Critical pathways as a strategy for improving care: Problems and potential. *Annals of Internal Medicine, 123,* 941–948.

Pravikoff, D. S. (2006). Mission critical: A culture of evidence-based practice and information literacy. *Nursing Outlook, 54,* 254–255.

Ramsey, S. D. (1999). Evaluating evidence from a decision analysis. *Journal of the American Board of Family Practice, 12,* 395–402.

Rashotte, J., & Carnevale, F. A. (2004). Medical and nursing clinical decision-making: A comparative epistemological analysis. *Nursing Philosophy, 5,* 160–174.

Sackett, D. L., Rosenberg, W. M. C., Gray, J. A. M., Haynes, R. B., & Richardson, W. S. (1996). Evidence-based medicine: What it is and what it isn't. *British Medical Journal, 312,* 71–72.

Sackett, D. L., Straus, S. E., Richardson, W. S., Rosenberg, W., & Haynes, R. B. (2000). *Evidence-based medicine: How to practice and teach EBM.* New York: Churchill Livingstone.

Schultz, A. (2005). Clinical scholars at the bedside: An EBP mentorship model for today. *Excellence in Nursing Knowledge, 2.* Retrieved September 15, 2006, from www.nursingknowledge.org/Portal/Main.aspx?pageid=36&Sender=Primary&SKU=51102

Shadish, W. R., Cook, T. D., & Campbell, D. T. (2002). *Experimental and quasi-experimental designs for generalized causal inference.* New York: Houghton Mifflin Company.

Slawson, D. D., & Shaughnessy, A. F. (2005). Teaching evidence-based medicine: Should we be teaching information management instead? *Academic Medicine, 80,* 685–689.

Stetler, C. (2001). Updating the Stetler model of research utilization to facilitate evidence-based practice. *Nursing Outlook, 24,* 559–563.

Stevens, K. R., & Staley, J. M. (2006). The quality chasm reports, evidence-based practice, and nursing's response to improve healthcare. *Nursing Outlook, 54,* 94–101.

Straus, S. E., & Sackett, D. L. (1997). Using research findings in clinical practice. *British Medical Journal, 317,* 339–342.

Tanner, A., Pierce, S., & Pravikoff, D. (2004). Readiness for evidence-based practice: Information literacy needs of nurses in the United States. Retrieved September 16, 2006, from http://cmbi.bjmu.edu.cn/news/report/2004/medinfo2004/pdffiles/papers/4770Tanner.pdf

Titler, M., Kleiber, C., Steelman, V., Goode, C., Rakel, B., Barry-Walker, J., et al. (1994). Infusing research into practice to promote quality care. *Nursing Research, 43,* 307–313.

Weinfield, J. M., & Finkelstein, K. (2005). How to answer your clinical questions more efficiently. *Family Practice Management, 12,* 37–41.

White, B. (2004). Making evidence-based medicine doable in everyday practice. *Family Practice Management, 11,* 51–58.

White, L. L. (2006). Preparing for clinical: Just in time. *Nurse Educator, 31,* 57–60.

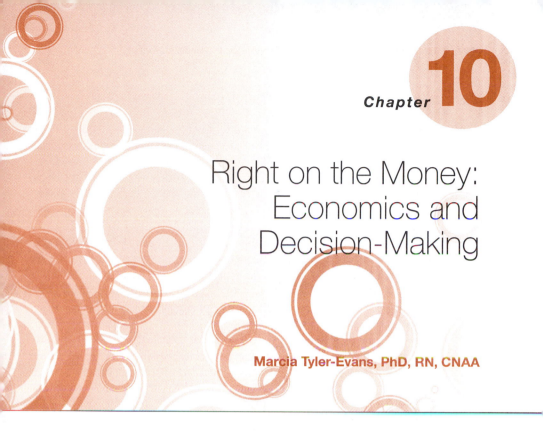

Marcia Tyler-Evans, PhD, RN, CNAA

Chapter 10

Right on the Money: Economics and Decision-Making

This chapter informs nurses and other health care professionals who work at the bedside and in the community about the important role economics plays in the health care decision-making process. In today's complex world, nurses must be aware of economics from both a macro- and micro-level. In particular, nurses need to know how to use this economically driven information as they make decisions and provide care within the environmental context that they are practicing. Nurses must understand, from a broad perspective, how the economy of health care as a whole is derived and driven. To this end, the nurse and all health care professionals must be aware of the relationships of this macro-level to the specific unit of practice known as microeconomics (McConnell, 2002). This chapter presents how economics on a macro-level influence the decisions nurses make on a daily basis. In addition, this chapter provides a micro-level view of economics and its effect on nurses' decision-making processes. A case study will highlight the use of an economic decision-making model in nursing.

Macro-Level and Decision-Making

Rising health care costs rivet our attention as one of the leading economic influences faced by the nursing profession. Health care costs use an increasing portion of the U.S. national gross domestic product (GDP). Henderson, Meyers, Ibrahim, and Tierney (2005) assert "health care is the public's third-highest priority after the war in Iraq and the economy" (p. 1062). Health care spending in the United States exceeds that of any other country. Henderson et al. (2005) project that during the next decade the proportion of the GDP spent on health care will reach approximately 20 percent. Their projections are based on current trends including health care insurance cost escalation by 60 percent since 2001, Medicare beneficiaries paying 17 percent more in monthly premiums between 2004 and 2005, and a prescription cost increase of 20 percent in the same period (Henderson et al., 2005).

Multiple forces are suggested to drive the escalation of the health care expense that include but are not limited to the following. First, Americans must acknowledge that most health care cost is indirectly paid for by the consumer. The majority of U.S. health care consumers participate in insurance or public health care coverage plans. The Medicare current beneficiary survey 1992–2002 reveals 79 percent of all health care costs are indirectly paid by private insurance or governmental programs. Only 21 percent of health care-related expenses are covered by individual out-of-pocket expenditure (CDC, 2002).

Second, Americans must consider that the overall population growth is contributing to the increase in expenditure for health care and in particular the cohort representing individuals 65 years of age and older who demonstrate the most rapid growth. Due to the advancing age of the largest cohort, the baby boomers, study projections published by the Center for Health Workforce Studies, School of Public Health at University of Albany in New York, suggest that between 2000 and 2020, the U.S. population will add 19 million older adults (Moore et al., 2005), thus adding a further strain on the health care system. With this growth, there is an expectation that there will be a higher volume of need for health care services. At the same time, while these same Americans are getting older, they are also getting sicker and more obese than in decades past. They expect the newest and best treatments and stand accused of overusing the health care system (Henderson et al., 2005). In addition, critical to this equation is the consideration that there is also a graying of the health care worker force and the projected shortages of key staff that will follow.

Third, public policy is another influential factor in rising health care cost. Some view government-enacted mandates such as the Health Insurance Portability and Accountability Act (HIPAA) as contributing to increased cost. Well-intended public policy mandates add complexity to an already overburdened system of health care delivery. Unfortunately, "policy-makers have not resolved the barriers to access and health insurance that deny care to at least 45 million Americans" (Woolf & Johnson, 2005, p. 546).

Not to be overlooked is the fourth and seldom-scrutinized contribution of the insurance "administrative sector." DeBakey (2006) asserts the number of insurance administrators expanded disproportionately to the number of physicians over the period between 1970 and 1995. DeBakey (2006) compares the 24 percent increase of U.S. physicians against the 2,000 percent proliferation of administrators over the same period. Finally, another component in the rising health care cost is malpractice premiums for organizations and professionals that encourage defensive and therefore more expensive health care. The 2002 Harris Poll in which physicians, nurses, and hospital administrators were asked about the impact of liability, 79 percent said that more tests were ordered than professional judgments deemed medically necessary (Garfinkel Weiss, 2005). Health care providers in this litigious environment order more extensive and expensive testing to assure their patients that all possible information was available for diagnosing their health problem (DeBakey, 2006). This testing pattern supports diagnosis and demonstrates exhaustive studies in the event a diagnosis is unclear or unpleasant. Considering all of these contributors to the rising cost of health care, Americans really must look at more than just the GDP as a measure.

Trends Affecting Economics

Economists project an increase in national health expenditures from current (DeBakey) level of $1.7 trillion to double by 2014, consuming $3.6 trillion (2006). The economic projection based upon a trend beginning in 1960 through today (DeBakey) suggests health care will drain as much as 25 percent of the nation's resources by 2030 (2006). The explosive growth in national health care costs is attributable to several trends, including an increasing population, an expansion of the elderly component which is projected to reach more than 45 million in the next 10 years, escalating administrative costs, and a costly advancement in medical technology, diagnostic equipment, pharmaceuticals, and surgical procedures (DeBakey, 2006). DeBakey further asserts that in 15 years, a projected 25 percent of federal income taxes will be used for Medicare (2006). Kaiser Family Foundation (2006) noted yet another trend. The total cost of all forms of individual health care continues to rise. Individual out-of-pocket expense has experienced an upward and downward cycle over the last 40 years in relationship to the national health expenditures (Kaiser, 2006). During this period, public and private efforts to rein in accelerating costs through wage and price controls, voluntary hospital cost containment, and most recently through managed care and the threat of health reform have triggered sharp declines in private spending growth. However, these periods of decline always have proven temporary and have been followed by rapid growth in costs. Average annual growth in private per capita health spending was 3.7 percent from 1960–2004 (Kaiser, 2006, p. 4).

Examining the various components of health care, the Kaiser Family Foundation identified the trends of spending and their changes in the most recent decade.

> While remaining the largest overall contributor to spending on health services, the proportion of national health expenditures devoted to hospital care declined from 34.1 percent in 1994 to 30.4 percent in 2004. At the same time the share spent on prescription drugs almost doubled from 5.6 percent to 10.0 percent of health spending in the U.S. (Kaiser, 2006, p. 5).

Meanwhile, physician and ambulatory clinic costs rose by 9 percent.

Changing Demographics

As noted earlier in this chapter, the U.S. population is aging. Projections for health care needs as the baby boomers approach retirement age are mixed. The baby boomers represent the largest cohort of working nurses. The boomers also represent two-thirds of all U.S. workers (Zemke, Raines, & Filipczak, 2000). By 2010, the "veteran generation," the individuals born between 1922 and 1945, will be 65 or older (Weston, 2006). This adds to the ever-growing elder population requiring health care. With advancing age of the general population, the United States is also experiencing a rise in the incidence of chronic illness. The most commonly occurring diseases revealed in the current medical literature include diabetes, hypertension, lung diseases such as asthma, cardiovascular diseases, and cancer. Many of these chronic illnesses are spurred on not only by age but modifiable risk factors such as diet, smoking, and exercise which many individuals neglect to integrate in their life via healthy choices.

For example, obesity is one of the many chronic illnesses that contribute to many of these diseases and thus the rising health care costs. Obesity is defined by the Centers for Disease Control and Prevention (CDC) as a person having a very high amount of body fat in relation to lean body mass, or body mass index (BMI) of 30 or greater. BMI is a measure of an adult's weight in relation to his or her height, specifically the adult's weight in kilograms divided by the square of his or her height in meters (CDC, 2006). Obesity trend data collected since 1990 reflects a gradual and unrelenting incline. In 1990, 11.6 percent of the U.S. population qualified as obese based on BMI. By 1991, only four states reported obesity prevalence rates of 15–19 percent and no states had rates at or above 20 percent. In 1995, obesity prevalence in each of the 50 states was less than 20 percent. By 2005, only four states reported obesity prevalence rates less than 20 percent, while 17 states had prevalence rates equal to or greater than 25 percent, with three of those having prevalence equal to or greater than 30 percent (CDC, 2006).

The rising incidence of obesity in the United States parallels the increasing frequency of diabetes type 2 (CDC, 2006). Individuals living with diabetes also demonstrate higher occurrences of coronary artery disease, peripheral vascular disease, major end organ damage such as renal failure, and blindness (Hogan, Dall, & Nikolov, 2003). The constellation of related medical problems associated with diabetes is associated with increased cost of health care. Therefore, obesity and diabetes represent a rising economic impact for the individual and the health care system. Changes, such as these, in the national demographics contribute to the unrelenting rising health care cost and drive the migrating health care delivery venue.

Health Care Delivery Changes Venue

Weinberg (2003) notes the transition from inpatient to outpatient services between 1983 and 1998. Weinberg's research cites American Hospital Association data claiming outpatient services doubled during the 15-year period while inpatient services remained flat or fell by as much as 10 percent, allowing for regional differences. These changes in patterns are reflected in the average length of stay (LOS) in U.S. hospitals. LOS declined from 7.2 days in 1981 to 5.5 days in 1996 (Weinberg, 2003).

Decreasing LOS impacts the character of the inpatient population in hospitals. The average medical-surgical patients in U.S. hospitals in the 1990s were as acutely ill as critical care patients in the 1980s (Curtin & Simpson, 2000). Presently these patients are discharged soon after they require less-intensive care and they must therefore seek the assistance of community health care providers, rely upon family or friends, or they must qualify for rehabilitation within a skilled care setting. The prevailing trend of shortened inpatient stay coupled with higher patient acuity boosts the patient care workloads for nurses in hospital settings. This increased patient care workload occurs in an environment of professional and skilled worker scarcity.

Health Care Resource Consumption and Changes in the Payment System

Health care resource consumption, as outlined in the chapter so far, diverts resources away from other programs and in so doing creates a strain on corporations that are attempting to provide workers, for example, with health care benefits. The outcome of this strain is the increasing need for individuals and families to increase their out-of-pocket expenses for health care services. U.S. citizens enjoy a health care system that is fundamentally job based, with nearly two-thirds of the nonelderly population receiving insurance as a job benefit (Lamb, 2004). The United States spends nearly twice as much on health care as any other of the 28 industrialized nations (Lamb, 2004). The Graham Center (2005) research trend analysis projects that annual health insurance premiums will exceed the average yearly household's income in 2025 if the present rate of escalation continues.

There have been many "cost-containment" efforts in the past but they have generally failed to reap their promised rewards. Attempts to restrain health care cost expansion began in 1973 with the enactment of the Health Maintenance Act (HMA). The Nixon administration instituted a "voluntary" freeze on health care spending initiated by the need to curtail health care spending during a period of double-digit inflation. Fee for service represented the primary method of payment between 1965 and 1983. By contrast, between the years of 1983 and 1998, implementation of the payment system based upon diagnostic-related groups (DRGs) and then prospective payment systems (PPS) and later resource-based relative value (RBRV) scales dominated health care reimbursement. Health care providers reeled under the stress of declining payments, hospital bankruptcies, massive deficits, layoffs, and merger dissolutions (DeBakey, 2006; Samuel, Raleigh, Hower, & Schwartz, 2003). Government efforts to constrain advancing consumption of national economic resources moved the health care reimbursement system from the open ended fee for service through the confines of DRGs to fully implemented managed care.

Restructuring Health Care Organization Generates Professional Shortages

Scarcity of professional and skilled workers sprang from hospital cost-cutting efforts in the late 1980s and lasting into the late 1990s. Responding to the changes in reimbursement, hospitals joined forces in purchasing networks as well as downsizing staff. Beginning with the management level, health care organizations flattened their organizations. The goal of decreasing personnel cost drove further reorganization efforts. Finding this insufficient to reduce the overall cost of care, restructuring, retooling, downsizing, and/or merger with other institutions, hospitals hoped to expand market share and reduce the overall organizational cost of care in relationship to reimbursement received. All of these changes were reflected in lay-offs affecting managers, nurses, and support staff. This period also witnessed a decline in health professions enrollment related to the challenges for employment in a shrinking job market. Retooling, product line creation, and realignment continued in the health care industry to ensure solvency and gain some kind of competitive advantage.

Restructuring took many forms in hospitals across the country. One of the most well published and publicized was patient-centered care (Parsons & Murdaugh, 1994). To their credit, the promoters of patient-centered care (PCC) believed the "health care delivery system was seriously flawed, suffering from escalating costs, variable quality, increasing bureaucracy and a lack of access" (Parsons & Murdaugh, 1994, p. xix). They proposed PCC as an opportunity to improve care delivery, decrease cost, and improve patient satisfaction. The foundation of PCC focused on placing multitasking care providers in the system to ensure the efficient overlapping of tasks intended to maximize productivity and minimize cost of delivery. The multitasking health care workers conceptually worked as nurse extenders, carrying out tasks such as serving meal trays, providing basic hygiene, ambulating patients, transcribing physician orders, and transporting patients, equipment, or specimens.

Parsons and Murdaugh (1994) asserted the new model of health care must be integrated, price sensitive, and value and health maintenance oriented to best serve the enrolled capitated populations. In capitated payment systems, a hospital or physician would be paid a fixed amount per member per month for all hospital or medical services which might be needed by a health maintenance organization's enrollees (DeMuro, 1995). Capitation is the health insurance method based on negotiated contracts with health care systems or individual providers to care for a specific population of clients for a fixed amount of funding per month. "Under fixed contracts, providers maximized their profit by limiting the number of contacts with patients and the quality of services provided" (Samuel et al., 2003, p. 121). Managed care limited access to control cost but patients responded demanding political intervention. Political interventions included the passage of the Patient Bill of Rights and easing of limitation of patient legal remedy for perceived failure to pay for needed medical services.

During this same time period in the early 1990s, the business environment in the United States embraced reorganizing, downsizing, restructuring, and reengineering to position their organizations in a highly competitive global environment. Hammer and Champy (1993) popularized the concept of and described the process of reengineering. Hammer and Champy (1993) as well as other "health care consultants" inspired enormous revamping of health care business structure for care delivery. Some hospitals viewed this model as an opportunity to reduce staffing expense. Adopting PCC and reengineering, hospitals restructured the workforce. In some health care restructuring efforts, nurses were "invited" to reapply for their job. Nurses faced job loss on a large scale, ultimately forcing nurses to pursue other options for practice or leave nursing all together.

The transition from inpatient care to outpatient care, as noted earlier, accelerated at this time. As a result, home health care agencies flourished. Outpatient surgical centers sprung up, attracting nurses away from acute care hospitals. Ambulatory care centers formed to provide renal dialysis and pediatric and diabetes care also needed nurses. Nurses accepted positions with insurance companies as case managers and as consultants for health maintenance organizations (HMOs) responding to member questions on nurse help lines. Reineck and Furino (2005) observed the migration of registered nurses (RNs) out of the acute care setting related to the movement of care into the community. Nurses drifted from inpatient to outpatient settings following the transition of health care services.

Supply and Demand of Health Care Worker Shortages

Immersed in an atmosphere of rising concern for patient safety, hospitals soon sought to augment their ranks of RNs. Hospitals faced obstacles attracting nurses back to care for increasingly critical patients. According to Sigma Theta Tau International's (1999) research on the nursing shortage conducted in 1996, the national vacancy rate of registered nurses in acute inpatient settings reached an all-time high of 20 percent. The U.S. Department of Public Health (DPH) noted the decline of available nurses. Dependent on baccalaureate-prepared nurses, in some practice environments, the DPH changed hiring criteria in some states. For example, in public health, a new category for public health nurses was added with the hope of attracting the associate degree–prepared nurses into the role of caring for clients in the community.

Supply side economics reveals concern about the aging nursing workforce and a diminished pipeline of new students entering the nursing profession due to broadening job opportunities within and outside of health care (Sigma Theta Tau International, 1999). Senator Mikulski (2001) quoted the findings of the subcommittee on aging in which 50 percent of the current nursing workforce will retire in the next 15 years (Mikulski in Wittmann-Price & Kuplenman, 2003). Reineck and Furino (2005) cited the American Hospital Association 2002 report addressing the rapid aging of the RN workforce, projecting escalating retirements in an era of increasing demand for nursing services. Furthermore, Reineck and Furino observed the "health care system characterized by scarce resources and increasing challenges of aging nursing and patient populations" impact the supply of working nurses (2005, p. 30).

Demand side economics demonstrates the number of hospitalized, critical, labor-intensive patients increased due to the aging population and medicine's success in keeping people alive longer, thus requiring more nursing hours to care for the increasingly complex patient population (Upenieks, 2003). Seifert (2000) observed that a key demand factor exemplified by the decrease in length of stay and the increase in acuity level of patients was never fully appreciated in cost-cutting equations. Clearly the health care environment must find balance between the supply side and demand side of this economic portrayal.

Health Care Safety

The new millennium ushered in a new awareness of health care worker shortages and health care safety concerns. Patient safety issues arose as public debate. Quality of care in the aftermath of all the downsizing and restructuring in hospitals came under public scrutiny in high-profile research study results. Research released in October 2002 demonstrated a relationship between hospital nurse staffing and patient mortality (Aiken, Clarke, Sloane, Sochalski, & Silber, 2002). A higher ratio of patients to nurses was linked to complications such as higher rates of internal bleeding, infections, and a higher risk of death according to a study published in the *New England Journal of Medicine* (Fischman, 2002).

Patient and nurse safety require attention as well. Patient safety relates to patient/nurse staffing ratios (P/N ratios). Research supports the relationship between the number of patients assigned to a registered nurse and patient care outcomes. Patient care outcome factors can include: Infection rates; falls; medication errors; and total number of inpatient days. Aiken et al. (2002) "found in hospitals with high patient-to-nurse ratios, surgical patients experience higher risk-adjusted 30-day mortality and failure to rescue rates and nurses are more likely to experience burnout and job dissatisfaction" (p. 1). Aiken et al., (2002) studied the cost-effectiveness of patient-to-nurse ratios ranging from 8:1 to 4:1. Further, they observed the patient data addressing mortality and length of stay revealed for every additional patient beyond four assigned to a nurse resulted in a 7 percent increase in the risk of death for each patient (Aiken et al., 2002). Decisions about the retention of qualified, experienced nurses at the bedside therefore become part of the economic equation as one factors the high cost of medical errors.

Retention of Professional Staff as an Economic Factor

American Hospital Association (AHA) research suggests a lack of positive, healthy work environment as one of the variables contributing to the nursing shortage (AHA, 2002). Considering the AHA findings, perceptible movement within the health care industry suggests movement toward cultural change. Efforts to align more closely with the criteria for "magnet status" gather momentum within the health care industry.

Magnet status is a designation achieved through the magnet recognition program. The magnet recognition program accredits hospital for nursing excellence that exhibit four critical elements: (1) management, philosophy, and practice; (2) integration of recognized quality improvement standards; (3) support for professional practice and continued nursing competence; and (4) understanding and respecting the cultural and ethnic diversity of patients, significant others, and health care providers (Stone, Larson, Mooney-Kane, Smolowitz, Lin, & Dick, 2006). Promoting cultural change to include these elements promises to help health care organizations to retain a valuable asset—nurses—and by collateral, benefit other valuable professionals and paraprofessionals.

Work environment includes additional factors such as relationships among management and administration, nursing peers, other professionals, patients, and families. Respect arises as a major factor in job satisfaction among nurses and thus retention. DeLellis and Sauer (2004) studied respect in health care settings and reported that 79 percent of those surveyed felt workplace respect was lacking in the United States to the extent that it was a serious problem. Respondents believed the quality-of-work life would improve if employees would care about and respect each other as much as they do their patients (DeLellis & Sauer, 2004). Rosenstein (2002) suggests, for example, that improving the quality of nurse-physician relationships can improve nurse recruitment and retention.

Nurse safety in health care settings relates to absence of physical injury. Nurses report nursing workload related to an increasingly aged, severely ill, and obese patient population add to physical and interpersonal stressors as a major concern. New issues emerge related to ergonomics in the workplace, thus effecting health care decision-making (Reineck & Furino, 2005). Nurses handling heavier patients and patients less able to assist themselves require more help and assistive devices to ensure the patient's safety as well as their own. Avoiding patient falls and staff injury goes directly to the hospital's net revenue in excess of cost. Therefore, promoting safety, providing lifting and moving devices, and sufficient professional and support staff pay dividends in lower-risk exposure, lawsuits, and workers' compensation claims. Patient and nurse safety are significant factors in the universe of improving the working environment and determining the care that is provided.

All the components contributing to the health care work environment–nursing job satisfaction and patient safety directly affect the economic bottom line of the health care organization. Turnover of health care staff is a significant factor in health care costs. Jones (2005) estimated the total turnover costs of one RN ranged from $62,000 to $67,000 depending on the service line. Turnover includes the cost of recruiting and in some cases, travel, housing, and sign-on bonus expense as well as finders' fees for recruiter. Additionally, orientation, proctoring/training, overtime replacement, and inefficiency during the learning phase of the new employee must be factored into the overall cost. The other side of turnover is the loss of experience and knowledge. According to Hatcher (in Barclay, 2006), lost knowledge not only impacts the bottom line but the "brain drain" can decrease innovation, increase costly errors, reduce efficiency, and undermine growth strategies. Hatcher's report of findings suggests that retaining older nurses is crucial to addressing the national nursing shortage, as well as the high cost of nurse turnover (Barclay, 2006).

Public Questions Corporate Profit Taking

The intent of managed care plans addressed cost containment. Unfortunately, most for-profit HMOs concentrate on substantial financial returns for investors rather than on quality and quantity of services. DeBakey (2006) cites data compiled by the *Wall Street Journal* disclosing that of the five top health insurance companies, annual income ranged from more than $5 billion to more than $20 billion with profits ranging from $352 to $935 million.

DeBakey (2006) asserts the backlash against HMOs now experienced in the United States reflects public disillusionment with the promises of low-cost, high-quality health care. All of the shifting of services, increased intensity of care in the acute care setting with a dilution of skilled professional nurses, discharging patient earlier back into the community, or transferring to a lower level of care failed to reduce overall health care cost as promised. The U.S. public now revolts against the restriction on access to care through the HMO insurance structure. Sensitive to public outcry, in 1998, Congress introduced legislation for patients' rights and some state legislatures accept patients' suits against HMOs (DeBakey, 2006). Subsequent suits alleging inappropriate denial of services and wrongful death against managed care insurers now successfully waged by patients or their family survivors change the relationship between the insurers and the insured. Publicity warning the U.S. public revealing a crisis of medical errors, highlighted cases of patient injuries, operations on the wrong limb, or worse yet the wrong patient receives a craniotomy. These sensational headlines cause public and political groups to ask questions. Fear of the health care system emerged. The U.S. health care system appears to be on the cusp of change again.

Applying Macro-Level Economics to Micro-Level Economic Decision-Making

"Restoration of a health care delivery system that is grounded in humanistic values and centered on patients' well-being is a contemporary challenge" (Donley, 2005, p. 317). Preventative care and patient education are at the forefront of systematic change. Engaging the client in a partnership for the purpose of managing their health in a cost-effective way is the direction nurses must lead. Contemporary nurses must implement health assessment and risk analysis in the broadest context to empower people to take personal responsibility for their health and health status (Donley, 2005). Nurses can accomplish health promotion and patient self-responsibilities in many health care venues.

Acute care settings like medical-surgical units, critical care units, ambulatory nursing centers, diagnostic testing services, specialty clinics, primary preventative health clinics, schools, outpatient surgery, cosmetic services centers, outpatient dialysis units, and public health practice with the needs of vulnerable populations in mind, all lend themselves to holistic nursing and client partnerships. Nursing care must be evidence-based and be ever mindful of the economics of decision-making.

The new health care delivery reality requires nurses to be educated as knowledge workers. Some of the opportunities available to nurses include clinicians, clinical specialists, teachers, clinical nurse leaders, clinical information specialists, clinical researchers, care coordinators, case managers, managers of complex care systems, practitioners, hospitalists, informaticists, collaboratists, consultants, and entrepreneurs. Specialty nursing demand for public health/community health nurses, critical care nurses, emergency room nurses, and focused specialties of cardiology/pulmonology, neurology, endocrinology, and trauma will flourish. However, again within these roles is the importance of economics in the nurse's daily decision-making.

Nurses face the challenge of articulating what they do, how they do it, where they do it, with whom they do it, and the cost of that care. Specifically, nurses must be prepared to link health care outcomes to specific best practice nursing actions inclusive of cost. Nursing actions must be qualified and quantified, thereby rendering those actions tangible with specific attached value. Nurses no longer have the luxury of ignoring cost. Nurses with knowledge of informatics can relate nursing actions with cost and thus play an important role in bringing nursing to the proverbial economic "table." It is for these reasons that all nurses, as health care professionals, must be aware of the broader terrain of the macro-economics of the time and how these broader issues affect and are affected by the micro-decisions made in daily practice. The following case is an example of this with a clear demonstration of the role of politics, economics, and policy.

The Context of the Case Study: The Macro- and the Micro-Level

A Macro Description

In 1988, the state of Oregon faced an unprecedented budgetary crisis related to a downturn in the general and local economy. Responding to the reality of fiscal shortfalls, the legislature altered the decision-making for allocating funds for basic health care for uninsured Oregonians. Legislators recognized health care–spending choices would be better made prospectively (Lamb, 2004). The Oregon plan's genesis sprang from necessity. Explicit health care rationing emerged and evolved as a strategy for providing basic health care services to a larger proportion of the uninsured or underserved in Oregon.

The Oregon plan demonstrated that a systematic model of explicit health care rationing can be implemented with grassroots input and high-level policy-makers involved. It defined a decent minimum level of health care, applying the utilitarian decision-making model, incorporating the general public values, and a cost-effective analysis ranking all medical interventions (Lamb, 2004).

The utilitarian decision-making model offers a straightforward model for deciding the morally right course of action. "The theory of utility generally defines 'good' as happiness or pleasure and 'right' as maximizing the greatest good and least amount of harm for the greatest number of persons" (Davis & Aroskar, 1983, p. 31). The opposition of "rightness" versus "wrongness" is also known as *calculus morality*, in which the argument considers the effect of alternative actions on the general welfare of present and future generations in a given situation (Davis & Aroskar, 1983, p. 31). The crafters of the Oregon plan operationalized this model, applying it to prioritizing health care services. Those services then were made available to the Oregon uninsured population.

The Oregon plan successfully expanded the population being served by limiting the content of care. Medicaid coverage extended to 130,000 poor Oregonians. As the Oregon plan was implemented, the proportion of uninsured persons fell from 18 percent in 1992 to 14 percent in 2002 (Lamb, 2004). The Oregon plan established a potential template for a national level program. Although a spirited debate continues in public and policy circles, universal health insurance is not an imminent reality. National, state, and private resource consumption remains a pressing issue.

A Micro Decision

The Oregon Health Plan (OHP) currently provides for such diverse populations as persons receiving therapy for symptoms related to human immunodeficiency virus (HIV) positive status and children with special health care needs (CSHCN). CSHCN is defined in a variety of ways including use of services, functional status, limitations in social role activities such as school or play, conditions or categories, or a combination of the aforementioned (Mitchell, Khatutsky, & Swignoski, 2001). CSHCN includes children with chronic and acute diseases such as asthma, appendicitis, retinopathy of prematurity, and spina bifida.

A study examined the impact of the OHP on children with special health care needs as compared to other groups covered by other funding agencies such as supplemental security income (SSI) or private managed care insurance (Mitchell et al., 2001). The authors found that children enrolled in OHP experienced greater difficulty obtaining services and gaining access to care than did those covered by SSI, a federally funded survivors program, or private managed care provider. These findings raise concerns regarding the efficacy of health care access for OHP-covered populations.

Examining this limited study outcome as an exemplar, how might this information be factored into nurse decision-making when advocating for patients covered by or qualifying for OHP? How does the nurse case manager interpret the regulations and health care inclusion/exclusion for persons with a specific diagnosis or fall under a specific category? Comparing the disease process, presenting symptomatology, and urgency of need against qualification for service and analyze the following case.

Application to a Case Study

A 32-year-old mother of three children makes application for coverage of the children for health care under the OHP. She is physically separated from her husband, living in a separate abode, with no intention for reconciliation. Her current status, however, requires that her husband's income be considered for the application. The husband has no insurance coverage available for the family's health care needs and has no real or personal assets. With his current income, the family does not qualify for OHP funds.

The youngest child, born prematurely, suffers from chronic asthma. The two older siblings each intermittently experience recurrent chronic otitis media. All of these health problems qualify for services under the OHP/CSHCN program but as stated, the husband has no insurance and his current income does not qualify the family for OHP. The mother is represented by an Oregon state welfare social worker who was assigned to this family and contacted you through OHP requesting consideration for covered services.

Considering the OHP/CSHCN program priority list, you know there are state funds to cover primary care for the children's health conditions reported by the social worker. As the nurse case manager, what action plan might you formulate with the social worker to provide some direction for this mother to qualify her children for health care services under the OHP? What obstacles might be anticipated when considering medical care coverage for this family? What might be the long-term cost of untreated chronic health conditions versus prevention and treatment by a primary-care provider? What is the cost-benefit ratio that having care versus not having care will generate? What are the costs of providing primary care for the children in this family versus cost of care when sought through the emergency services system? How would you construct a proposal of care to the CSHCN program medical director? Nurses must ask these kinds of questions when making decisions about care. Economics of care factor into the decision and knowing what questions to raise are important to the decision-making process.

Here are some of the ways in which a nurse can respond to the questions just raised. The first step is to instruct the mother regarding the importance of establishing legal separation and filing of the divorce petition (this establishes the family's financial vulnerability). Legal standing is a huge obstacle for this family. Without the formal legal petition filing for separation and divorce, the family is considered dependent to the father. Even though the family does not receive any financial support from the father, that income is still considered. The second step is that the mother must provide information regarding the family's current living arrangements and an accounting of expenses to determine the level of need in relationship to the available funds versus health care costs (this helps to document level of need). In the third step, you must have the mother document the health care history of each child including all immunizations to date to identify the starting point for program needs (this information serves as a foundation for understanding previous patterns of care and real expenses). Fourth, a plan for primary health maintenance and wellness care for all three children must be developed. Cost out the expected visits, interventions, and medications necessary for your plan to be implemented and carried out for one year (this establishes a comparison against which to measure the value of care received and projected).

For the fifth step, project a cost-benefit analysis (CBA) based on previous interventional care and a plan for primary health maintenance care for each child. The CBA and cost effectiveness refer to a formal comparing of the negative and positive consequences of a project or investment (Finkler, 1994; Finkler & Kovner, 2000). As Finkler (1994) states, CBA is often shrouded in technical jargon and mathematics, however, the process is really nothing more than attempts to weigh logically the pros and cons of a decision. Compare the projected cost of continued interventional care including any emergency care visits from the previous year against your proposed health maintenance plan for each child. In the sixth step, develop a formal proposal based on the existing standard of care for each diagnosis using the OHP references. The CBA is the centerpiece of the proposal. Remember to include a one-page, single-spaced case and proposal summary as a face sheet. Send a copy in advance to the OHP medical director with a cover letter of explanation. Finally, schedule an appointment with the OHP medical director to discuss the case, taking a copy of the proposal and summary as well as the case file with you.

Conclusion

The health care drain on the United States economy was explored from the macro perspective measured by the GDP consumption of approximately 14% and climbing each year. Public policy and insurance administration influence on the rising cost of health care were examined. Changing demographics of the general population as well as that of the health care providers were considered for their contribution to the advancing expense of providing health care to the citizens of the country. The increasing incidence of chronic diseases was also reviewed. The health care environment and escalating cost are multi-factoral.

The economic environment in which health care is delivered in the United States can not be ignored. Nurses must understand the significance of the macro level economic issues and how they influence the micro level of decision making in clinical practice. Mannion, Small, and Thompson (2005) assert that the "power of economic ideas shapes the discourse of nursing and through this influence the choices and activities of nurses" (p. 370). Nurses can influence as well as be influenced by the realities of health care economics. Nurses must apply the macro economic view to the micro economic setting in daily clinical decision-making.

References

Aiken, L. H., Clarke, S. P., Sloane, D. M., Sochalski, J., & Silber, J. H. (2002). Hospital nurse staffing and patient mortality, nurse burnout and job dissatisfaction. *Journal of the American Medical Association, 288*(16), 1987–1993.

American Hospital Association Commission on Workforce for Hospitals and Health Systems. (2002). *In our hands: How hospital leaders can build a thriving workforce.* Chicago: American Hospital Association. Retrieved August 11, 2006, from www.aha.org/aha/research-and-trends/health-and-hospital-trends/2006.html

Barclay, L. (2006). Retaining older nurses in hospital practice: A newsmaker interview with Barbara J. Hatcher, PhD, RN, MPH. *Medscape Medical News 2006.* Retrieved August 11, 2006, from www.medscape.com/view article/537115

Centers for Disease Control and Prevention, National Center Health Statistics. (2002). Personal health care expenditures of Medicare beneficiaries by source of payment, type of services, sex, race/ethnicity, residence and age, from the Medicare current beneficiary survey 1992–2002. U.S. Department of Health & Human Services. Retrieved August 11, 2006, from www.cdc.gov/209.217.72.34/aging/TableViewer/tableView.aspx

Centers for Disease Control and Prevention, National Center Health Statistics. (2006). State-specific prevalence of obesity among adults— United States, 2005. *Morbidity Mortality Weekly Report, 55*(36), 985–988.

Curtin, L., & Simpson, R. (2000). Staffing and the quality of care. *Health Management Technology, 21*(5), 42–45.

Davis, A. J., & Aroskar, M. A. (1983). *Ethical dilemmas and nursing practice* (2nd ed.). Norwalk, CT: Appleton-Century-Crofts.

DeBakey, M. (2006). The role of government in health care: A societal issue. *The American Journal of Surgery, 191,* 145–157.

DeLellis, A., & Sauer, R. (2004). Respect as ethical foundation for communication in employee relations. *Laboratory Medicine, 35,* 262–266.

DeMuro, P. R. (1995). *The financial manager's guide to managed care & integrated delivery systems: Strategies for contracting, compensation & reimbursement.* New York: Irwin Professional Publishing.

Donley, R. (2005). Challenges for nursing in the 21st century. *Nursing Economics, 23*(6), 312–318.

Finkler, S. A. (1994). *Essentials of cost accounting for health care organizations.* Gaithersburg, MD: Aspen Publications.

Finkler, S. A., & Kovner, C. T. (2000). *Financial management for nurse managers and executives* (2nd ed.). Philadelphia: W.B. Saunders.

Fischman, J. (2002). Nursing wounds: When arrogant docs drive nurses away, patients suffer. *U.S. News and World Report, Health & Medicine, 132*(21), 54.

Garfinkel Weiss, G. (2005). Malpractice: How fear changes practice. *Medical Economics.* Retrieved May 17, 2005, from http://www.memag.com/memag/article/articleDetail.jsp?id=154646&searchString=How%20fear%20changes%20practice

Graham Center. (2005). *Who will have health insurance in 2025?* Retrieved July 20, 2007, from http://www.aafp.org/afp/20051115/graham.html

Hammer, M., & Champy, J. (1993). *Reengineering the corporation: A manifesto for business revolution.* New York: HarperCollins.

Henderson, M. C., Meyers, F. J., Ibrahim, T., & Tierney, L. M. (2005). Confronting the brutal facts in health care. *The American Journal of Medicine, 118*(10), 1061–1063.

Hogan, P., Dall, T., & Nikolov, P. (2003). Economic costs of diabetes in the U.S. in 2002. *Diabetes Care, 26*(3), 917–932.

Jones, C. B. (2005). The costs of nurse turnover, Part 2: Application of the nursing turnover cost calculation methodology. *Journal of Nursing Administration, 35*(1), 41–49.

Kaiser Family Foundation. (2006). *Trends and indicators in the changing health care marketplace.* Retrieved September 22, 2006, from www.kff.org/insurance/7031/print-sec1.cfm

Lamb, E. J. (2004). Rationing of medical care: Rules of rescue, cost-effectiveness, and the Oregon Health Plan. *American Journal of Obstetrics and Gynecology, 190*(6), 1636–1641.

Mannion, R., Small, N., & Thompson, C. (2005). Alternative futures for health economics: Implications for nursing management. *Journal of Nursing Management, 13*(5), 377–386.

McConnell, B. (2002). *Economics.* New York: McGraw-Hill Irwin.

Mikulski, B. A. (2001). In R. Wittmann-Price, & C. Kuplenman (2003). A recruitment and retention program that works! *Nursing Economics, 21*(1), 35–38.

Mitchell, J. B., Khatutsky, G., & Swignoski, N. L. (2001). Impact of the Oregon health plan on children with special health care needs. *Journal of the American Academy of Pediatrics, 107,* 736–743. Retrieved November 11, 2006, from www.pediatrics.org/cgi/contents/full/107/4/736

Moore, J., Salsberg, E., Wing, P., Dill, M., McGinnis, S., Stapf, C., & Rowell, M. (2005). *The impact of the aging population on the health workforce in the United States.* Albany, New York: University of Albany, Center for Health Workforce Studies, School of Public Health.

Parsons, M. L., & Murdaugh, C. L. (1994). *A model for restructuring.* Gaithersburg, MD: Aspen Publishers.

Reineck, C., & Furino, A. (2005). Nursing career fulfillment: Statistics and statements from registered nurses. *Nursing Economics, 23*(1), 25–30.

Rosenstein, A. H. (2002). Nurse-physician relationships: Impact on nurse satisfaction and retention. *American Journal of Nursing, 102*(6), 26–34.

Samuel, T. W., Raleigh, S. G., Hower, J. M., & Schwartz, R. W. (2003). The next stage in the health care economy: Aligning the interests of patients, providers, and third-party payers through consumer-driven health care plans. *The American Journal of Surgery, 186,* 117–124.

Schwenk, T. L. (2002). Low nurse staffing ratios, patient safety, and nurse burnout. *JournalWatch.* Retrieved October 1, 2006, from http://general-medicine.jwatch.org/cgi/content/full/2002/1108/1

Seifert, P. C. (2000). The shortage. *Association of Operating Room Nurses Journal, 71*(2), 310–312.

Sigma Theta Tau International. (1999). *Facts on the nursing shortage.* Indianapolis, IN: Author.

Stone, P. W., Larson, E. L., Mooney-Kane, C., Smolowitz, J., Lin, S. X., & Dick, A. W. (2006). Organizational climate and intensive care unit nurses' intention to leave. *Critical Care Medicine, 34*(7), 1907–1912.

Tucker, B. (2006). National Labor Relations Board announces new ruling, it forbids workers from joining unions if they perform so-called supervisory duties at work. Atlanta, GA: CNN. Retrieved October 5, 2006 from http://www.Loudobbs.com

Upenieks, V. (2003). Recruitment and retention strategies: A magnet hospital prevention model. *Nursing Economics, 21*(1), 7–13.

Weinberg, D. B. (2003). *Code green: Money-driven hospitals and the dismantling of nursing*. New York: Cornell University Press.

Weston, M. J. (2006). Integrating generational perspectives in nursing. *Issues in Nursing, 11*(2), 1–7. Retrieved on August 11, 2006, from http://www.medscape.com/viewarticle/536479

Wittmann-Price, R., & Kuplenman, C. (2003). A recruitment and retention program that works! *Nursing Economics, 21*(1), 35–38.

Woolf, S. H., & Johnson, R. E. (2005). The break-even point: When medical advances are less important than improving the fidelity with which they are delivered. *Annals of Family Medicine, 3*(6), 545–549. Retrieved August 11, 2006, from http://www.annfammed.org/cgi/reprint/3/6/545?maxtoshow=&HITS=10&hits=10&RESULTFORMAT=&author1=Woolf&andorexactfulltext=and&searchid=1&FIRSTINDEX=0&sortspec=relevance&resourcetype=HWCIT

Zemke, R., Raines, C., & Filipczak, B. (2000). *Generations at work: Managing the clash of veterans, boomers, Xers, and nexters in your workplace*. New York: AMACOM.

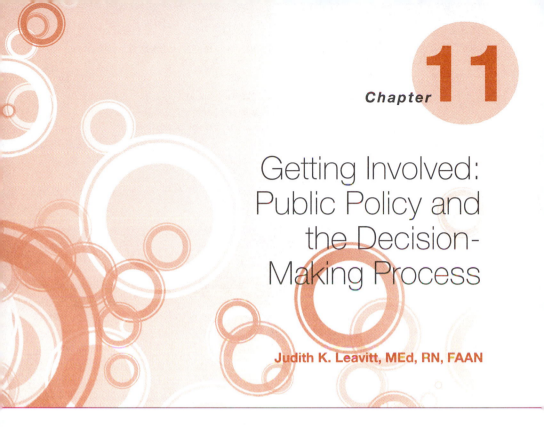

Chapter 11

Getting Involved: Public Policy and the Decision-Making Process

Judith K. Leavitt, MEd, RN, FAAN

What is public policy and why do nurses need to use the information in helping clients? At first glance, it seems like a curious connection, yet so much about the work of nursing involves decisions and influences beyond the nurse–client relationship. Think about how many patients are denied or limited in their care because of third-party payment, private or public insurance. What about the elderly client who is unable to get needed medication because the drug is not included on the formulary of their Part D Medicare plan? And what about the nurse practitioner (NP) who must give up caring for a particular patient because the NP is not included as a preferred provider in the patient's new health plan? These are real issues that most advanced practice nurses will confront. Decisions around such issues involve public policies that affect practice. The policies and the leverage that the nurse has to respond involve the political environment. One must ask if the laws and regulations enable a nurse to practice to the full extent of her or his ability or do such laws and regulations place significant restrictions on practice? If the answer is that they do not, then the process of lifting such restrictions means that nurses and the profession must engage in political action to advocate for supportive health policy.

Certainly there is precedence for such involvement as noted by Lewenson (2007). Our foremother, Florence Nightingale, was one of the first to argue for the need to change the larger sociopolitical environment to improve health—and the concept of sociopolitical knowing was reinforced in Carper's classic 1978 work as crucial to practice.

Policy, Politics, and Values

Mason, Leavitt, and Chaffee (2007) use a framework to discuss the interaction of policy, politics, and values that provide an understanding of how to incorporate knowledge about the policy and political arena in decision-making. What is policy? *Policy* is defined as "principles that govern action directed towards given ends" and as a choice of action to achieve a particular goal (Titmus, 1974, p. 23). In public policy, it is the choices that the public and policy makers make about issues that affect the populace. Policy choices reflect the values of those who make the policies, the policy makers, who in turn are affected by the group being served (Mason et al., 2007, p. 3). *Politics* involve the influences used to achieve the goal and always involve groups or individuals with different kinds of power; in other words, the groups with the most power and influence (be it resources, money, people, or connections) are going to be most successful in getting what they want.

All politics and policy take place within a particular value system. For instance, NPs who advocate to prescribe medications as school nurses are assuming that parents and decision-makers support and value this role for advanced practice nurses (APNs). The way that value system may be expressed is through supportive regulations that enable the APN to independently prescribe medications for children enrolled in a nurse-managed school health center.

Another example is allowing NPs to treat minors for a sexually transmitted disease. If the predominant values of state legislators oppose minors receiving care without parental permission, then nurses will be unable to provide such care in that state. Unless nurses are aware of the predominant values of the public and policy makers around a particular issue, it may be fruitless to advocate a course of action, such as trying to get supportive legislation, which is in opposition to prevailing values.

The Policy Process

As part of ways of knowing how to resolve an issue, it is often vital to know whether there are laws and regulations that impede effective practice and if so, what they are. Therefore, to understand public policy, one must know how government works and how to exert political influence to get supportive policies.

How Government Works

As you remember from high school civics class, there are three branches of government: executive, legislative, and judicial, and three levels of government: local, state, and federal. Health policy is made by all three branches and at all three levels of government. For instance, practice issues are usually made at the state level. State legislatures pass laws that define a Nurse Practice Act and state Boards of Nursing develop the specific regulations that give definition to the general outline of the law. For example, in New York state, the definition of the Nurse Practice Act in Article 139, section 6902 reads:

> The practice of the profession of nursing as a registered professional nurse is defined as diagnosing and treating human responses to actual or potential health problems through such services as case-finding, health teaching, health counseling, and provision of care supportive to or restorative of life and well-being, and executing medical regimens prescribed by a licensed physician, dentist or other licensed health care provider legally authorized under this title and in accordance with the commissioner's regulations. A nursing regimen shall be consistent with and shall not vary any existing medical regimen. (New York State Nurse Practice Act, 2006)

The law gives only the outline of nursing practice. The regulations spell out what is meant by case finding, health teaching, and prescribing. The same section of the New York law defines nurse practitioner practice. Here is an excerpt:

> The practice of registered professional nursing by a nurse practitioner, certified . . . may include the diagnosis of illness and physical conditions and the performance of therapeutic and corrective measures within a specialty area of practice, in collaboration with a licensed physician qualified to collaborate in the specialty involved, provided such services are performed in accordance with a written practice agreement and written practice protocols (New York State Nurse Practice Act, 2006).

It is the Board of Nursing (or in New York, the State Department of Education) who define regulations like the "collaborative agreement." For instance, it would identify what the collaborative agreement must include, who can sign it, and how long it is effective. If the law states, as it does in New York, that an NP must take a pharmacology course to qualify for writing prescriptions, the regulations would define the kind of pharmacology course required to have prescriptive authority.

At the federal level, the Medicare law (Title XVIII of the Social Security Act) defines that an NP can be reimbursed for services. However, the regulations of Medicare, which are promulgated by the Centers for Medicare and Medicaid (CMS) under the U.S. Department of Health and Human Services, will define exactly which services would be covered.

Even the judicial branch of government influences health policy, primarily through enforcement of legislative and regulatory requirements. However, it is when these laws and regulations are challenged that the judicial system has the greatest impact. At the federal level, one of the most controversial decisions was *Roe v. Wade* in 1973. That decision, based on various amendments to the U.S. Constitution, upholds the right of a woman to make decisions about her own body. This interpretation thus conferred a woman's right to choose an abortion, if she so wished. Even though subsequent challenges have occurred with states placing more restrictions on abortions, the original decision still stands.

Federal Government

Washington, D.C., is the center of federal government where the legislative branch, Congress; the executive branch, the president and his or her cabinet; and the judicial branch, the Supreme Court, reside. The legislative branch consists of the two houses of Congress: the House of Representatives and the Senate. The House has 435 seats apportioned as a result of the U.S. Census, which is taken every 10 years. The number of seats in a particular state may vary depending on the number of residents in a state but the total number in the House will always equal 435. House members are elected every 2 years, in November of an even numbered year.

The Senate has 100 members; two from each of the 50 states. Terms of office are 6 years. Approximately one third of its members are elected every 2 years. The political party with the majority of seats is known as the *majority* party for that calendar term (which is the 2-year term when members of the House of Representatives are elected).

The majority party elects a leader, who in turn, appoints chairs of all the committees. This enables the majority party to have considerable political power in determining which legislation is introduced as well as which bills move through committees for a vote.

The primary role of the legislative branch is to make laws. Legislation is introduced by an elected member of Congress (at the federal level) and assigned to the committee in that house with jurisdiction over the issue. Legislators from each chamber often introduce the same bill simultaneously. Only a senator can introduce a bill in the Senate and only a member of the House can do the same in the House of Representatives. There are approximately 250 committees and sub-committees to examine the bills and hold hearings. In each session thousands of bills are introduced. Only a few make it through the complete process to implementation.

The majority leader in each house will determine which committees will have jurisdiction over the bill. Once a bill is introduced and sent to a committee, the chairperson will decide if and when hearings on the bill are held and what changes can be made before the bill is voted on by the originating committee. Often bills, such as those involved with health care, must be acted on by more than one committee. For instance, if a particular bill at the federal level concerns Medicare, it would be considered by both the Energy and Commerce Committee as well as Appropriations Committee. Though having different committees consider a bill can enable lobbying by more advocacy groups, it also slows the process toward passage or defeat. If a particular piece of legislation has money attached, it will have to be considered by the Appropriations committees in each house. Members of the subcommittees on Health of the Appropriations committee have a significant role in allocating revenue for each legislative proposal. For a fuller discussion of the appropriations and authorization process, see Hendrickson and Cohen (2007, pp. 680–684).

The same bill must be approved by majority vote in both houses of Congress and signed by the president to become law. If a bill is voted down at the committee level or passed by only one house, the bill is considered "dead." Also, if it makes it through both houses of Congress but is vetoed by the president, it will not become law. The only way it could pass after a veto is if both houses override the president's veto with a two thirds majority. Few laws are passed in this way and usually only after the president has lost considerable power.

Executive Branch

The president, as the chief executive of the federal government, is responsible to oversee the implementation and enforcement of federal laws. Through the cabinet officers and numerous agencies, commissions, and committees, the president creates regulations that define federal laws. For health providers, one of the most significant is the U.S. Department of Health and Human Services (HHS) and its 12 operating divisions with over 300 programs. These include everything from Medicare and Medicaid, to CMS, to drug enforcement, the National Institutes of Health, and the Public Health Service. (See the department's Web site at www.hhs.gov/about/index.html.) The HHS provides funding for nursing education as well as defines reimbursement policy under Medicare. It also provides some federal mandates for Medicaid and the State Children's Health Insurance Program (S-CHIP).

Other important federal agencies involved in health care include the U.S. Department of Defense which administers military health programs, the Veterans Administration, and the Departments of Education and Labor. Information about each is easily accessible online to determine federal standards, accountability, and program opportunities.

The power of the executive branch at the federal level emanates from the president's role in appointing cabinet secretaries with Senate approval. Because each serves under the direction of the president, department policies reflect the president's political and policy agendas. The other power of the president is in his or her ability to sign or veto legislation, particularly if his or her party has enough votes in Congress to sustain a veto.

Judicial Branch

The courts at the federal level have jurisdiction over matters that involve the U.S. Constitution and federal laws and regulations. The highest court is the U.S. Supreme Court, arbiter of last resort. There are 94 district courts where most federal cases originate. There are 11 federal appeals courts as well as two circuit courts. Though not traditionally thought to make policy, the judiciary branch has in fact been defining health policy through its decisions. For instance, the federal courts are increasingly becoming involved in labor disputes and medical liability issues, as well as issues of right to life and right to die (see Betts, Keepnews, & Gentry, 2007). Legal scholars expect this trend to continue as states and federal governments create public policies related to privacy, liability, and public funding of health programs.

State Government

The structure of the state government is the same as the federal with several differences. All states except one, Nebraska, have two houses in the legislature, called *bicameral* legislatures. They may have a variety of names for their state legislatures, such as general assembly, legislative assembly, or the general court, but all are responsible for making state law, confirming governors' appointments, and approving state budgets. Most meet every year though a few meet every other year (Montana). Some have a defined timeline, like a 3-month session (Mississippi) and others meet throughout the year, like California. State legislatures have jurisdiction over licensing and practice acts, most educational policies and funding, welfare and work programs, and numerous health programs, including public health and school health. Medicaid and S-CHIP are federal/state programs though states have increasing authority over the programs. The regulatory responsibility of the states is to develop rules around many of these issues, including nursing practice and the rights of patients.

Governors serve as the chief officer of states. More than half have lieutenant governors, the second in command, who may or may not be a member of the same political party as the governor. The power of the governor varies and is determined by the state constitution. However as more decision-making has devolved from the federal level to the state (devolution) governors and state legislatures have increasing power to determine policy. All governors have the responsibility to propose a state budget and manage the budget after it is approved by their legislatures. They also have veto power over legislation. One of the most important political powers a governor has is to appoint heads of departments as well as governing boards who develop the regulations. One example is the Board of Nursing. In some states, certain department heads may be elected or appointed by one of these governing boards; thus the governor can influence the process through the appointment of the people he or she selects for governing boards. As a result, administration in power can have considerable power over nursing practice.

Local Government

If it is true that all politics is local, the local government, because it is closest to the people, is the easiest to influence. The third level of government, the local level, has a variety of organizational structures and influence on health issues. Much is dependent on size. For instance, large U.S. cities, such as New York, Los Angeles, and Chicago, have city governments that are as complex as many states. It may administer its own Medicaid program as well as have considerable autonomy over public health. Most have jurisdiction over many aspects of public health, school policy, water and sanitation, and police and fire. Local governments administer school health through either local school boards or through public health departments.

The structure of governance can vary greatly from counties with elected boards like board of supervisors, or through a single individual, the county executive or county manager. It is essential to know how your local government works to know how to influence health policies (see Mason, 2007, pp. 685–687).

Influencing the Process: Political Action

It is vital to know how government works and how public policy is made but such knowledge has limited effect unless one knows how to influence the policy makers who make the laws and regulations that support patients and nursing practice. To have influence means to have power; to understand how to influence, one must determine who has power, what kind of power, and the extent of power in relation to others. Nurses and patients have power if they learn how to use it effectively. This is the essence of advocacy. (For more about power and political analysis, see Leavitt, Cohen, & Mason, 2007, pp. 77–86.)

Political Strategies

Political strategies provide the guidelines for decision-making and action. Strategies are most effective when carefully planned and done with groups of people. Rarely does an individual have enough power to influence a policy outcome. Working in coalitions with others who represent different constituencies, advocates can be more powerful in affecting policy. It takes persistence to keep policy makers focused on the issue. The most successful advocates are those who have a long-standing relationship with policy makers and can call upon them and keep them informed on a regular basis, not just at a time of crisis. For nurses, that means getting to know your legislators and representatives before you need them. Share your expertise about health issues. Invite them to your place of employment to understand the needs of your clients. When they get to know you, they will be more responsive when you ask for their help.

Legislation can take time to pass and be implemented. At the state level, it usually takes at least 3 years to pass. At the federal level, it can take much longer; for instance, the Family and Medical Leave legislation took 18 years.

Persistence also requires that you offer solutions to issues, not just identify problems. Policy makers are rarely experts in health.

Consider these strategies for action:

- **Be prepared.** Be well informed on the issues, including knowing the perspectives of different constituencies, especially the opposition. It enables you to prepare policy makers to respond to alternative arguments.
- **Frame the issue appropriately.** Place your issue in a larger context. For instance, if the issue is about insurance reimbursement, frame the issue as an "access to care" solution.
- **Work with others, preferably through coalitions.** Broad support for an issue assures a policy maker that they are taking the popular stand that reflects constituent support.
- **Know the goal—and be willing to compromise.** No legislation or regulation is ever agreed to without considerable changes.
- **Assess the timing for action.** Be sensitive to the larger political and policy environment to know when to "push" for an issue. If the values of the public and the policy maker conflict with your issue, it might be best to move slowly in the beginning until there is congruence on the issue. However, always be prepared for a "full-court press" if it looks like there is support for the issue.

The bottom line is that the best health policy is only as good as the ability to get it implemented. That is the heart of political action.

Case Study 1

School Nurses: A Local Issue

Betsy Stand is a school nurse in a rural county of Mississippi. She covers four elementary schools with over 1,500 children. Because of the distance between schools, she spends one full day at each school and then divides the fifth day amongst the different schools. One of the policy issues that she confronts is medication administration. She knows as an RN how important it is to know about each medication, each child receiving it, and the need to do an assessment both before and after administration. However, the school board has allowed secretaries and teachers to give the medications because the school nurse is not present when many of the medications must be given. Betsy had two events in the last month in which children had adverse reactions to the medications. One occurred because a wrong dose was given; the other because the medication had been discontinued, but the information was not given to the teacher who administered it.

Betsy needs to make a decision about how to handle the issue. How should she proceed?

Step 1. Assessing the Problem. Betsy checks the medication policy and determines that it was developed by the school district; however school nurse policy is developed by the Mississippi State Board of Nursing. She knows the Board is the regulatory agency for practice and any policy changes have to be approved by the full board. Members are appointed by the governor, usually with nominations from state nursing organizations.

Step 2. Information Gathering. Betsy checks the Board of Nursing Web site for new regulations and then calls both the state nurses association and the state association of school nurses. She shares the problem and asks for their suggestions and help in devising a policy that is safer for the child, is realistic, and is cost effective. Both nursing groups agree to help find a solution for the problem.

Step 3. Developing a Plan. Betsy asks for a meeting of nursing groups to develop a medication policy. Attendees included the executive director of the Board of Nursing, the president of the school nurse association, and the executive director of the state nurses association. They developed three different options to give medications: the teacher, a licensed practical nurse (LPN), or the RN. A grid was created to look at the costs, available personnel, and the chances of support and opposition for each. It was agreed that the most cost-effective, realistic option would be to recommend each school hire an LPN who would be required to take a prescribed medication course. She or he would be supervised by the RN who was responsible for that school. Though there would be an increase in cost for the school, the group was prepared to show that the cost would be offset by safety concerns for the students and decreased liability from potential medication errors.

Step 4. Gaining Support. The three agency directors agreed to meet with the state Department of Education and the school board association about the issue. Betsy was to meet with the president of the local school board to apprise her of the potential policy change. Most agreed to the suggested change and were able to convince their colleagues to support the change. The executive director of the Board of Nursing then shared the information with the other board members. School nurses across the state were asked to send letters of support to state board of nursing members prior to their vote.

Step 5. Implementation. The vote was passed and the policy approved. Betsy and other members of the school nurses association worked on local implementation policies in each school district. LPNs were hired and after 1 year, there were no medication errors in any school district in the state.

Case Study 2

APRNs as Network Providers: A State Issue

Roger Warren is a family nurse practitioner who has been in practice for 5 years. His patient Sam has taken a new job with the state and is now getting health insurance through the state employees' health plan. Roger called to check if he was a preferred provider and found out that nurse practitioners were not covered. What should he do to get this policy changed?

Step 1. Assess the Problem. Roger called the plan administrator to find out why NPs were not covered and how such decisions about preferred providers were made. He was told that the governing board of the plan made the decisions and that the governor appointed the individuals to that board. Members included private citizens and state employees but one third were state legislators. Because the legislature had to pass the budget for the state employee health plan, Roger knew the legislators on the governing board would have considerable power over the legislature's budget and therefore over fiscal policy for the state participants.

Step 2. Information Gathering. Roger decided to call the state NP network to find out if they had ever tried to get deemed status. He was told that in fact there was an attempt 5 years earlier that was unsuccessful. The NPs tried to get the regulation changed but had done so as individuals rather than with organizational support. In the meantime, the NPs were seeing patients under the auspices of their collaborating physician and patients were billed at the physician rate. Roger knew that this was illegal and could jeopardize the practice of both NPs and their collaborators. He was told that there was considerable support for NPs in the legislature and that the NP network was ready to organize an effort to change the rules. He also checked with the state board of nursing to see if there was anything to prevent their moving forward. He was told that in fact the NPs should do so because they were in jeopardy of committing fraud, if they were billing inappropriately. The state nurses association indicated strong support and help in working on the issue.

Step 3. Developing a Plan. The groups decided that the first person to visit was the chair of the Health Committee in the House of Representatives. He was a legislator who had been very responsive to nursing concerns, more so than the chair of the health committee in the state senate. The purpose was to learn who the legislators were on the governing board of the state health plan, whether the chair would support reimbursement for the NPs, and whether he would work with resistant colleagues to garner support for the NPs. Because the legislature had to approve the budget for the state health plan, it was critical that the leaders supported the NP's request. The chair indicated his willingness to help.

Step 4. Implementation. A group representing the NPs and the state nurses association met with each legislator who was on the governing board, as well as the chair of the board and the plan administrator. Information was shared about the cost effectiveness and outcomes for NPs. They requested the same payment rate as that used for Medicaid, which was legislated to cover NPs at 90 percent of the physician rate. They shared information about NP outcomes for Medicaid patients, all of which were as good, or better, than physician outcomes. The administrator expressed strong support and promised to share the information with the board. Two months later, the board voted approval with a defined credentialing process for providers interested in applying.

These examples provide a framework for how nurses can develop decisions about practice issues that require knowledge about public policy and political strategies to affect positive outcomes. In both situations, the nurse sought help and support from organizations that had an interest in the issue as well as extensive knowledge about legislation and regulations. For the individual nurse, the most important decision was recognizing what needed to be changed and working with others to make it happen.

Conclusion

This chapter focused on the ways in which public policy can inform nurses' decisions. Nurses who are knowledgeable about the political process and who are active in the political arena use information about public policy to influence the policy makers to appropriate decisions affecting practice. The interconnectedness amongst policy, politics, and values was explored. The reader was presented with a short synopsis of how government works to form a basis for understanding how to affect public policy. Strategies for influencing policy makers were presented and two case studies provide examples of how nurses can use knowledge about policy and politics to support nursing practice and patient care.

As this book illustrates, decision-making for the nursing practice is a complex process that requires knowledge about many fields, which often includes health policy. As we begin to incorporate this in our work, we will find that outcomes not only improve patient care but can expand our practice. It is empowering to know one has influenced legislation or regulation and even more so when seeing the benefits in improved health outcomes.

References

Betts, V., Keepnews, D., & Gentry, J. (2007). Nursing and the courts. In D. Mason, J. Leavitt, & M. Chaffee (Eds.). *Policy and politics in nursing and health care* (5th ed.). St. Louis, MO: Saunders/Elsevier.

Carper, B. (1978). Fundamental patterns of knowing in nursing. *Advances in Nursing Science, 1,* 13–23.

Hendrickson & Cohen, S. (2007). How government works and what you need to know to influence the process. In D. Mason, J. Leavitt, & M. Chaffee (Eds.), *Policy and politics in nursing and health care* (5th ed., pp. 680–684). St. Louis, MO: Saunders/Elsevier.

Leavitt, J., Cohen, S., & Mason, D. (2007). Political analysis and strategies. In D. Mason, J. Leavitt, & M. Chaffee (Eds.). *Policy and politics in nursing and health care* (5th ed.). St. Louis, MO: Saunders/Elsevier.

Lewenson, S. (2007). A historical perspective on policy, politics and nursing. In D. Mason, J. Leavitt, & M. Chaffee (Eds.). *Policy and politics in nursing and health care* (5th ed.). St. Louis, MO: Saunders/Elsevier.

Majewski, J., & O'Brien, M. (2001). Local government. In D. Mason, J. Leavitt, & M. Chaffee (Eds.). *Policy and politics in nursing and health care* (4th ed., pp. 487–489). St. Louis, MO: Saunders.

Mason, D., Leavitt, J., & Chaffee, M. (2007). Policy and politics: A framework for action. In D. Mason, J. Leavitt, & M. Chaffee (Eds.). *Policy and politics in nursing and health care* (5th ed.). St. Louis, MO: Saunders/Elsevier.

New York State Nurse Practice Act. (2006). Accessed November 2, 2006, from www.emsc.nysed.gov/sss/Laws-Regs/Health_Services/ Nurse_Practice_Act-full.htm

Titmus, R. M. (1974). *Social policy: An introduction.* New York: Pantheon.

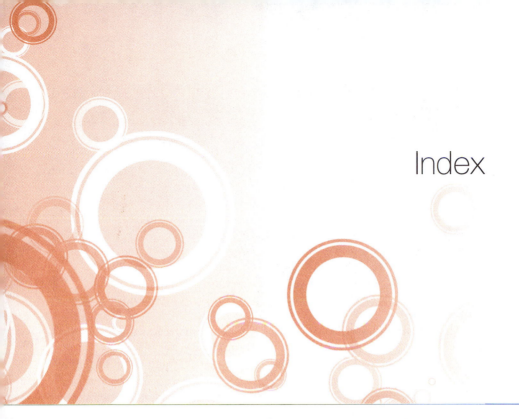

Index

Italicized page locators indicate a figure; tables are noted with a t.